Trances People Live

By turning the usual notion of trance on its head, Stephen Wolinsky has developed a revolutionary way of exploring how we create the trance states we live in, and how we can restore our freedom to live in present time. I believe this work has the ability to once again reform the way we understand ourselves. It is a major step towards replacing therapy with the potential of human learning.

Carl Ginsburg, Ph.D.,
Former President of the Feldenkrais Guild
and editor of *The Master Moves.*
Author of *Medicine Journeys: Ten Stories*

Trances People Live

Healing
Approaches In
Quantum Psychology

Stephen Wolinsky, Ph.D.

In collaboration with
Margaret O. Ryan

THE
BRAMBLE
COMPANY
Connecticut

For information write to:
The Bramble Company, RFD 88, Falls Village, CT 06031

ISBN 0-9626184-1-1 (Cloth)
ISBN 0-9626184-2-X (Paper)
Library of Congress Catalog Card Number: 91-72049

First Printing 1991
1 3 5 7 9 10 8 6 4 2

Printed in the United States of America

This book is dedicated to

The memory of Milton H. Erickson, M.D.

To Kristi, my love

And to Margaret O. Ryan,
whose invaluable collaboration
has made this book possible.

Acknowledgments

There are many who have contributed to my Ericksonian training and growth as a therapist over the years:
Paul Carter, Ph.D., Stephen Gilligan, Ph.D.,
Stephen Lankton, M.S.W., Carol Lankton, M.A.,
Eric Marcus, M.D., Nisargadatta Maharaj,
Braulio Montalvo, M.A., Bill O'Hanlon, M.S.,
Jack Rosenberg, P.D.S., Ph.D., Ernest Rossi, Ph.D.,
Neil Sweeney, Ph.D., Kay Thompson, D.D.S., and
Jeffrey Zeig, Ph.D.

Special thanks to my workshop participants and sponsors, whose support, love and participation infuse this book.

The Authors

Stephen Wolinsky, Ph.D., began his clinical practice in Los Angeles, California in 1974. A Gestalt and Reichian therapist and trainer, he led workshops in Southern California. He was also trained in Classical Hypnosis, Psychosynthesis, Psychodrama/Psychomotor, and Transactional Analysis. In 1977 he journeyed to India, where he lived for almost six years studying meditation. He moved to New Mexico in 1982 to resume a clinical practice. There he began to train therapists in Ericksonian Hypnosis, N.L.P. and family therapy. Dr. Wolinsky also conducted year-long trainings entitled: Integrating Hypnosis with Psychotherapy, and Integrating Hypnosis with Family Therapy. Dr. Wolinsky is currently working on a second book, *Quantum Consciousness: The Discovery and Birth of Quantum Psychology: The Physics of Consciousness.* He is the co-developer of Quantum Seminars™ and the founder of Quantum Psychology™. Along with Kristi L. Kennen, M.S.W., he founded the first Quantum Psychology Institute™. For more information write or call: Quantum Psychology Institute, c/o Dr. Stephen Wolinsky, Star Route Box 277, Placitas, New Mexico 87043, (505) 867-9392.

Margaret O. Ryan is a writer and editor in Los Angeles, California. She is co-editor (with Ernest L. Rossi) of the four-volume series, *The Workshops, Seminars, and Lectures of Milton H. Erickson.* She is also the collaborating author of *Therapeutic Metaphors for Children and the Child Within* (Joyce Mills and Richard Crowley), and editor of Carl Whitaker's *Midnight Musings of a Family Therapist.*

Contents

Foreword

To INCLUDE enough humor to make the reading enjoyable, to be autobiographical in a way that lends intensity and legitimacy, and finally, to present both the studious quality and the thinker quality is a massive bit of coordinated fullness.

In *Trances People Live* Dr. Wolinsky has made a unique project of combining his six years in the Far East studying their world with his 20 years as a therapy student studying our world. This unique integration makes his background for writing about Ericksonian psychotherapy, historic psychotherapy. Add to this some Eastern philosophy as well as Western religion and physics, and you've got a fascinating piece of literary choreography.

In *Trances People Live* the author presents a new conceptual framework for trance which translates into a comprehensible, psychotherapeutic, organized way of looking at daily life as a process of trance. Very exciting. His concept of everyday psychology as a process of self-induced trance is a wonderful way to begin. He is almost saying that trance is a new word for feelings. It is also a new word for the residuals of our life history.

As he moves from this point to a larger understanding and explanation of experiencing oneself as the context for one's feelings, he finds an intriguing way of teaching others how to experience the transformational insight that "I am not my problem." His understanding of the move from intrapersonal trance to interpersonal trance is a delightful extrapolation from the beginning premise that

"I am entranced by myself." He not only makes it clear that symptoms are an extrapolation within the context of self-hood, or I-hood, or person-hood, but goes from there to a perspective of the psychotherapy experience that includes the therapist's person-hood. Dr. Wolinsky's concept of the integrity of the therapist and his belief that the therapist-patient identity is a unity, and that the therapist's interpersonal honesty and freedom to express himself is central to his own beingness, makes the quality of this book a transcendent experience.

I loved reading *Trances People Live*, I highly recommend it, and please don't be confused by the word *hypnosis*. Dr. Wolinsky is talking about life.

Carl Whitaker, M.D.
March, 1991

Prologue

TRANCES PEOPLE LIVE was originally taken from transcripts of ongoing advanced Ericksonian hypnosis training seminars I was conducting in 1985. A year later I experienced a leap in my understanding of consciousness and the intrapsychic phenomenon called "Deep Trance." This leap continued an evolutionary process which culminated in the discovery and creation of Quantum Psychology and the founding of the first Quantum Psychology Institute in 1987.

It is difficult now, in 1991, to pinpoint any one event that triggered these new understandings. I could point to 23 years of involvement in the field of psychology. I could point to an 18-year meditation practice along with living in a monastery in India for almost six years. I could also consider my years of reading and researching in the area of Quantum Physics. Ultimately, my understanding was neither a culmination nor a cultivation created by some aligned cause and effect. Rather, it felt like a natural unfolding of who I was.

From 1987 to the present, the creation of the Quantum Psychology Institute™ became more possible through the planning, consultation, research, experimentation, and development with my partner, Kristi L. Kennen, M.S.W.

Although *Trances People Live* does not stress the concept of Quantum Psychology in depth, it does implicitly suggest and discuss one of the most important discoveries of Quantum Physics:

Heisenberg's "Uncertainty Principle." Nick Herbert, noted physicist and author of *Quantum Reality: Beyond the New Physics,* has called Werner Heisenberg "the Christopher Columbus of Quantum Physics"—the discoverer of the new, unchartered world of quantum physics amidst the well-worn pathways of the old world of Newtonian physics. Heisenberg forever changed the world of physics through his research which showed that the instrument of measurement as well as the observer of the experiment influence the outcome. According to Herbert (1985), Heisenberg's single finding has given rise to an array of philosophical interpretations within the scientific community, which he identifies as eight different schools of thought. One of these, the "Copenhagen interpretation," is the centerpoint of Quantum Psychology. Herbert (1985) explains that:

> The Copenhagen interpretation properly consists of two distinct parts: (1) There is no reality in absence of observation; (2) observation creates reality. You create your own reality is the theme of Fred Wolf's *Taking the Quantum Leap.* (p. 17)

In amplifying the Copenhagen interpretation of Heisenberg's Uncertainty Principle, Fred Wolf (1981) cites another physicist's view:

> Eugene Wigler, Nobel prize-winner in physics, believes that our consciousness alters the world itself, because it alters how we appraise the future. That is, we experience the world the way we do because we choose to experience it that way. (p. 211)

Wolf speculates: "How could there be a mechanical universe out there if the universe changed every time we altered *how* we observe it?"

Because of the active influence exerted by the observer in this Quantum universe, quantum theorist John Wheeler has added a significant refinement by changing the word *observer* to *participator*, stating that "no elementary phenomenon is a real phenomena until it is observed" (Herbert, 1985, p. 18).

Translated into Quantum Psychological terminology, this means that how we subjectively experience events, interactions, and our own inner self is observer-created—created *by us*. This reality suggests a further one: that we, as the knowers of our experience, choose how an experience is experienced. This is the pivotal entry point of Deep Trance Phenomena, the medium in which our creative activity takes place whereby we select how experiences are perceived, interpreted, and understood.

Throughout *Trances People Live: Healing Appraoches In Quantum Psychology*, the phenomena of hypnotic trance is viewed as a self-generated, self-created reality that appears to happen *to* us. In fact, we discover that each self-created reality is comprised of a specific Deep Trance Phenomenon (or clusters of several Deep Trance Phenomena) that results in what we typically refer to as symptoms or problems. Acknowledging our observer-created trances—trances created by us—begins a deeper process of assuming responsibility for the part we all play in creating (however unknowingly or unconsciously) our own hypnotic and phenomenological realities. The task of the therapist becomes one of observing and identifying the self-generated problem state or hypnotic trance and *de-hypnotizing* the person out of the trance he or she is already in.

Most therapists and psychotherapy theorists believe that there is an interpersonal feedback loop that takes place in every experience. For the most part, however, we go inside ourselves and construct our own meaning of events, quite independent of what "actually" occurs. For example, if I say, "I like you," you might create any number of responses: (1) "That's nice"; (2) "He didn't really mean it"; (3) "If he only knew what I was really like, he'd never feel that way"; (4) "I wonder what he wants from me."

All these responses—which are also trances—are self-generated and happen "automatically" as we move from what appears to be an *inter*personal loop (self-to-other) to an *intra*personal loop (self-to-self). Understanding that the Deep Trance Phenomena we use to create our problems and symptoms are observer-created sets the stage for de-hypnosis and lays the groundwork for a new Quantum Consciousness unbounded by the limitations of our current conception of "reality."

Stephen Wolinsky, Ph.D.
New Mexico, 1991

1

A Day In The Life Of A Trance

SIX YEARS AGO I had a breakthrough moment that changed the way I did therapy and brought together 15 years of study in Eastern and Western traditions. While working with a woman whose presenting problem was alcoholism, I suddenly realized that she was spontaneously creating her own trance phenomena, and that *it was those very trance phenomena that made her symptom of excessive drinking possible*. I then began to notice that all the symptoms my clients presented had at least one Deep Trance Phenomenon associated with them. I was particularly surprised to note that in order for a symptom to remain a symptom, there had to be at least one Deep Trance Phenomenon that the person created to hold the symptomatology together "like glue." Without the associated Deep Trance Phenomenon, *the symptom could not repeat itself*. In some cases, the Deep Trance Phenomenon *was* the symptom itself.

I had been trained to use trance work in the Ericksonian framework in which trance is seen as a special but natural state of consciousness that is optimally suited for mediating therapeutic work. Hypnosis is used as a means of bypassing the conscious mind and inducing (or "facilitating") trance so that problem resolution can take place on an unconscious level.

As I worked with my alcoholic client, I experienced a startling reversal of that understanding: now I saw trance phenomena as being *the means by which symptoms are created and maintained*. Trance was at the core of the symptom structure and thus at the core of symptom relief. In the next few days another reversal took place in my understanding: what was currently being called "therapeutic trance" in the hypnotherapy community was really similar to the *no-trance state* in which a person's perceptions and observations flow unobstructed in the Eastern practice of meditation.

It was not necessary to induce or facilitate trance work in the therapeutic session, since the person arrived with her symptom — which meant that *she arrived with the Deep Trance Phenomenon that was being used to hold the symptom together*. By working with the symptomatic trance the person had already created, she would "pop into" a no-trance state (currently called "therapeutic trance") in which the symptom could be rapidly relieved. Furthermore, the job of the hypnotherapist was no longer to *induce* a trance but rather to *de-hypnotize* the individual out of the trance she was already experiencing. In short, there was no reason to create another trance to counter the symptom; rather, it was simpler and easier to utilize the trance (symptom) the client brought to the session.

In the remainder of this chapter we will explore a new, more comprehensive view of the experience of trance that goes beyond Erickson's concept of the "common everyday trance." We will see how Deep Trance Phenomena are at the core of a wide spectrum of experience that spans the symptoms, identities, roles, and reactions we create as adults. In Chapter 2 we will look at the etiology of trance as symptom as it is created and maintained in the early family environment.

Trance as Symptom

Let's explore a few everyday examples of trance states that underlie common problems to clarify this paradigm shift.

Anxiety is a fear of the future. A client whose presenting

problem is anxiety might be using a cluster of Deep Trance Phenomena to synthesize the sensation of anxiety. First comes *pseudo-orientation in time* as she imagines a catastrophic outcome occurring in the future and therefore experiences fear. Next she uses *posthypnotic suggestions* ("It will never work out," "I can't cope with life," "Nothing will help") to articulate and differentiate the particulars of the negative outcome she is imagining. These are reinforced by *negative hallucinations*, which block her ability to see or acknowledge other resources, and perhaps vivified by *positive hallucinations* as she visualizes herself encountering an anxiety-provoking stimulus (such as a bill collector) that is not present in present time. All of this turmoil is likely to be further exacerbated by an experience of *time distortion* in which she has a breathless feeling that there is not enough time to find any kind of solution.

Erickson (Erickson, Rossi, & Rossi, 1976; Erickson & Rossi, 1979) wrote about the "common everyday trance" that naturally occurs throughout the day. This is the type of light trance state that we all experience periodically. It is not particularly problematic and, indeed, it can even be refreshing. Driving along in the car, I hear a tune from 20 years ago and spontaneously age regress to a particular experience that is linked in my memory with that tune. Or, I am sitting in my favorite chair absorbed in a basketball game on TV and somehow manage not to hear a word that is said to me by my wife. Or, I look up from my desk where I have been hard at work for the past hour and glance outside, staring into the sky and the trees in a daydreamy, absorbing moment.

These examples of Erickson's common everyday trance involve a non-symptomatic and transitory use of Deep Trance Phenomena. In addition to these kinds of light trance states that Erickson described and utilized in his work are *trance states that function at the core of the symptom structure*. As we will see in Chapter 2, these kinds of trances are created by the child in response to threat and *become* sources of pathology as they are integrated into the child's habitual mode of response. By the time we reach adulthood, we have intricate patterns of defense woven out of clusters of Deep Trance Phenomena that appear to function autonomously within us. *Choice* becomes the key factor in ascertaining whether the trance we are in is part of the problem, part of the solution, or just a pleasant, refreshing experience. Am I locked into (identified with) this moment of dissociation? Or can I easily return my focus of attention? Am I choosing to experience pseudo-orientation in time, or did it seem to happen *to* me?

For example, as I am sitting in a restaurant listening to a friend talk, I find that something he has said about a recent movie has triggered associations in me: various pictures "pop up" automatically in my mind's eye, as I slip into recalling a similar movie I saw with an old girlfriend. I can let my mind continue to wander (that's one kind of trance state), or I can consciously choose to focus more intently on my friend (that may be another kind of trance state) — but either way, I am not in the grip of a problematic trance state over which I have no apparent control. A problematic trance would occur if I found myself slipping into a rapid depression as my wandering associations popped up painful memories from the past relationship (age regression), and I virtually stopped hearing or seeing my friend and the environment in present time (negative auditory or visual hallucinations) as I became "lost" in my ruminations. In both cases I am in a trance, but in the latter I can choose to move out of it or alter it easily, while in the former I become identified with it and its contents.

Trance as a Continuum

In the Eastern tradition we are seen as being trapped in "maya," the transient world of the mind. We identify with (and thus *become*) this transient inner world of thoughts, feelings, emotions. The entrapment comes not from the external sensate world per se, but from our identification with it and attachment to it. We identify with this feeling and that thought, we think we are no more than the bundle of sensations currently capturing our field of attention. These identifications and attachments create limitations which cause us much "suffering."

In a sense, trance states are transient and hence states of *maya*. These are states during which we narrow and constrict our attention (and our sense of selfhood) by identifying with our thoughts, feelings, and emotions in a manner which seems to be autonomous — rather than recognizing that we are the *knower* of these trance states, which are *transient*. We actually go in and out of trance states all day long, far more often than is commonly recognized. We experience a continuum of trance states — some pleasant, many not — in which we chug along in a bumpy series of identifications and attachments.

What is exciting about recognizing and *experiencing* the multitude of trance states we create throughout the day is that it leads to a transcendent experience of oneself. Each trance state has a *beginning* point, a *middle* point, and an *end* point. As you begin to step outside of your trances by identifying these component parts, what you begin to see is that the only common factor behind the series of trance states is *you*. There is a you, or a self, or a higher self that is outside of, or larger than, the comings and goings of these trance states. In addition, this *you* or *self* is creating the trance states — the trance states are not autonomous at all. By experiencing the step-by-step process we go through to create our trances (and, hence, our symptomatology), we automatically take control over them, which in turn enables us to go beyond them.

It is widely recognized that trance is characterized by a narrowing, shrinking, or fixating of attention. Erickson and Rossi (1976/1980) note:

> Trance is a condition wherein there is a reduction of the patient's foci of attention to a few inner realities; consciousness has been fixated and focused to a relatively narrow frame of attention rather than being diffused over a broad area. (p. 448)

To induce a trance state, hypnotherapists attempt to induce this narrowed foci of attention that is the core characteristic of trance (Erickson & Rossi, 1979):

> The fixation of attention has been the classical approach for initiating therapeutic trance, or hypnosis. The therapist would ask the patient to gaze at a spot or candle flame, a bright light, a revolving mirror, the therapist's eyes, or whatever. As experience accumulated, it became evident that the point of fixation could be anything that held the patient's attention. Further, the point of fixation need not be external; it is even more effective to focus attention on the

patient's own body and inner experience. . . .Anything that fascinates and holds or absorbs a person's attention could be described as hypnotic. We have the concept of the common everyday trance for those periods in everyday life when we are so absorbed or preoccupied with one matter or another that we momentarily lose track of our outer environment. (p. 4)

Another core characteristic of trance is the experience of it as happening *to* the person. In their five-stage paradigm of the dynamics of trance induction, Erickson and Rossi (1979) note that stage five, that of the "hypnotic response," is "an expression of behavioral potentials that are experienced as taking place autonomously" (p. 4). And, in a table entitled, "Some Common Indicators of Trance Experience," they list "autonomous ideation and inner experience" at the top of the list (p. 11). Gilligan (1987) elaborates:

> Experience in trance "just happens," without the regulation, control, or other active participation by self-conscious processes. . . .this characteristic of effortlessness is described by the principle of ideodynamicism, which states that ideas can be expressed in dynamics (sensations, images, cognitions, motor acts, perceptions, emotions) without any conscious mediation. (p. 40)

Finally, trance is characterized by the spontaneous emergence of various hypnotic phenomena (Erickson & Rossi, 1976/1980):

> Depotentiating a patient's usual everyday conscious sets [via trance] is thus a way of depotentiating facets of his personal limitations; *it is a way of deautomatizing an individual's habitual modes of functioning so that dissociation and many of its attendant classical hypnotic phenomena (e. g., age regression, amnesia, sensory-perceptual distortions, catalepsies, etc.) are frequently manifest in an entirely spontaneous manner.*" [Italics added] (p. 448)

We have now accumulated three core characteristics of trance:

1) trance is characterized by a narrowing, shrinking, or fixating of attention;

2) trance is most often experienced as happening *to* the person; and

3) trance is characterized by the spontaneous emergence of various hypnotic phenomena.

Keeping in mind these three core characteristics, let's explore the vast arena of trance states we experience that are not commonly identified as such.

In the course of any one particular day, you might experience what I would call a "beach trance," a "phobia trance," a "cute-kitty trance," and a "fight trance," to single out but a few.

Say you go to the beach on a Saturday, having completed a rough week of high-pressured work. You lay down, you "space out," you stare at the water, you feel the hypnotic warmth of the sun on your body, and you are generally having a wonderful time relaxing in the sand and sun (*beach trance*). Then some friends show up and you all go for a walk along the water's edge. Everyone begins roughhousing and you get pushed into the water. Unbeknownst to your friends, you are phobic about actually being in the water, and you begin to panic and feel like you are drowning (*phobia trance*).

You survive this ordeal, pack up and begin to walk home, whereupon you come across a teenager trying to give away several kittens. You stop dead in your tracks, pick up one of the kittens and begin talking like a five-year-old. You are so enchanted by the kitten that you spend 30 minutes there, talking "kitty-talk" and being completely oblivious to the time (*kitty trance*). You get home and promptly get into a fight with your partner in which you both scream and yell for 30 minutes because you were late (*fight trance*). Then you make up and cuddle, kiss, and tell each other how much you love one another for an hour (*love trance*).

There are two common factors in all of these trance experiences. The first is that each one had a *beginning* point, a *middle*, and an *endpoint* — which means that *you are the one common factor in the comings and goings of these particular trances.*

The second is that *each trance state* (be it a "pleasant" one such as going to the beach, or an "unpleasant" one such as getting into a fight) *was comprised of a cluster of Deep Trance Phenomena.* If you were to videotape your experience at the beach, you would probably be able to pinpoint the *trans*formation that came over you. When you first arrived, your body was tense and your movements were very focused; even your facial expression was still furrowed from the week. As the beach *happens to you*, you begin to "melt" into a mellow, unfocused state — lying on the sand, baking in the warmth of the sun, listening to the rhythmic splash of the waves. Without giving it a single conscious thought, the beach experience appears to have created in you a hypnotic state of relaxation filled with Deep Trance Phenomena such as time distortion, dissociation, anesthesia, sensory distortion, and so forth.

Perhaps you have a more active beach experience of running along the water, playing ball with a nearby child, laughing and splashing "like a kid again." When asked, "How was your day?" you might well answer, "Great! I felt like a kid again!" Basically, the beach environment has triggered an age-regressed state that appears to happen *to* you. After all, you didn't go to the beach with the conscious intention of creating an experience of playing like a kid again. Yet *you* did create that experience.

The *phobia trance* is comprised of an onslaught dose of *age regression* wherein you are thrown back in time to when, as a very young child, you got knocked down by waves and felt like you were drowning. Hand-in-hand with this time traveling is an experience of *pseudo-orientation in time* wherein you move forward in time to the imagined moment of catastrophe; and you experience an agonizing sense of *time distortion*: suddenly, time feels as if it is standing still and you are frozen in the grip of your panic. Next, "waves" of *posthypnotic suggestions* ("I might die!... Get me out of here. . .I'm a bad boy for being here. . .I'm going to die!") wash over your thoughts to complete your single-pointed experience of fear.

The *kitty trance* helps restore you to a more comfortable state. This time, your experience of *age regression* is a totally pleasant one as you slip back to those magical moments you had getting your first kitty. The narrowing of your focus of attention to the kittens is a pleasure to feel and contrasts sharply with the narrowing of your focus of attention to the state of panic you experienced (created) earlier. Similarly, your altered experience of time in the kitten trance (*time distortion* in which time is experienced as passing quickly) contrasts with the sense of time passing inexorably slowly in the panic trance.

The *fight trance* whips into motion through a swift kick of *age regression* to the tantrum age. You both yell and scream; one of you slams a book down for emphasis; the other turns his/her back and pouts. The tantrum then gets articulated and elaborated through a barrage of *posthypnotic suggestions* fired back and forth. Your partner shouts: "You're always late. . . you're never considerate of me. . . you only think of yourself. . .being late means you don't really love me."

You retaliate: "You're always *rigid*. . .you're never spontaneous. . .you only think of your *schedule*. . .if you loved me, you'd give me more *space!*"

Pseudo-orientation in time then takes your partner through the day in lightning speed and brings him/her to the unhappy conclusion that "the rest of the day is ruined!" Your conclusion is similar. You both march off to separate rooms, stewing in a trance that indeed creates the rest of the day (pseudo-orientation in time to the future) as being ruined in present time.

At last you both get bored by the stalemate and begin to talk things through. As the anger dissipates and sweet feelings arise, the *love trance* glides into motion. Your mutual age regressions of the tantrum phase now transform into the *age regression* of the powerless, dependent, grateful child phase. You both slip into baby-talk as you apologize, telling each other, "I love you," and proclaiming that, "You're the only person in the world for me," or, "I would be devastated without you," or "I'm more myself with you than with anyone else in the world" (*posthypnotic suggestions*). You both reassert your couplehood (*identity trance* — more on that later) and take comfort in your internal pictures of walking down the street together hand-in-hand, being responded to as a couple in restaurants, sharing one credit card and buying household items together (*pseudo-orientation in time*).

You may also experience some degree of *time distortion* in your love trance as time seems to stand still or disappear entirely.

This is not to say that all our moments of love are encumbered by trance states that take the experience out of present time and burden it with "unfinished business." However, such "pure" experiences of love (in Hindu literature it is called *prem*; in Western culture it is currently referred to as "unconditional love") are fairly rare. Most of us are more familiar with the intrusion of any number of psychodynamic "games" and "hang-ups" the moment we move into intimate, sustained contact with another person. The raw material of these games and hang-ups is Deep Trance Phenomena.

Table 1
The Deep Trance Phenomena comprising the continuum of trance experiences in the course of a day.

BEACH TRANCE
- age regression
- anesthesia
- dissociation
- sensory distortion
- time distortion

PHOBIA TRANCE
- age regression
- posthypnotic suggestion
- pseudo-orientation in time
- time distortion

KITTY TRANCE
- age regression
- time distortion

FIGHT TRANCE
- age regression
- posthypnotic suggestion
- pseudo-orientation in time

LOVE TRANCE
- age regression
- identity trance
- posthypnotic suggestions
- time distortion

Reactions as Trance States

Reactions are trance states when they happen *to* us — which is more often than not. We blow up, raise our voices, slam our fists down on table tops, get red-faced, get passionate. We don't usually experience ourselves as consciously, intentionally creating our reactions, especially when any degree of emotional valence is involved. We react back and forth in response to one another, which means, in essence, that we are creating trances that bounce back and forth.

Our own responses are valuable tools. As soon as we blurt out the reaction, we can see it clearly and become less identified with it. An example of reaction as trance can be seen in the familiar experience I call the "I Love You Trance." You are beginning a relationship, and it is going well. There is a lot of compatibility, the right amount of passion, and so forth. One evening, under the glow of a romantic moon, your partner says, "I love you."

We have all had various encounters with this declaration. Sometimes we are thrilled and begin to spin fantasies of an ecstatic life (*pseudo-orientation in time* and *positive hallucination*); sometimes we are anxious and begin to dread the inevitable breakup (*pseudo-orientation in time* and *positive hallucination*); or we may just feel a sense of pressure and contraction as we begin to obsess over, "What does this mean? Should we live together? How much time should we spend together? Are we a couple now? Should I tell her/him my daily schedule???" (*pseudo-orientation in time, post-hypnotic suggestion, age regression*).

From an enjoyable, in-the-moment experience, we suddenly move into one which creaks and struggles beneath structures of reactions. In essence, we are recreating the past in present time via various Deep Trance Phenomena. As we saw in a previous section, these trance phenomena "shrink-wrap" our focus of attention, leaving a very constricted perspective with which we usually strongly identify.

I had a client who arrived one day for a session red-faced and fuming. Jack immediately launched into a tirade about the event that was "causing" his distress.

It seems that he had submitted a proposal to his boss that he had hoped would result in a promotion. He had worked very hard on this proposal and felt it was "perfect" by the time he submitted it. His boss' response was mixed: Jack was told that much of it had value but that one of the key concepts struck him [the boss] as "meaningless" because it was not delineated well enough.

It was clear that Jack had not heard one word past *meaningless*. This word had instantly triggered a trance identity we later labeled as "No one ever gets me." Jack had then suffered predictable emotional distress as a result.

I asked Jack to recreate the experience in our session. He described how he had felt prior to receiving his boss' feedback: confident, even expansive, and excited. During the feedback, Jack's attention quickly narrowed to the word *meaningless* and he promptly *age-regressed* to all those childhood experiences with his father, with his teachers, with his peers — all of them "not getting me." A chain of prior events, all linked by the common *trance identity* experience of "No one ever gets me," was automatically activated by a certain word. One moment Jack was in an expanded state in which his work was going well; the next moment, with the utterance of those few words, he had flipped into a contracted state of anger, resentment, and hopelessness. This unpleasant state was comprised of a cluster of Deep Trance Phenomena that drastically narrowed his field of attention and his very sense of selfhood.

Symptoms and problems are the outermost manifestations of a creative, generative interaction of Deep Trance Phenomena. Once the clusters of Deep Trance Phenomena that coalesce into symptoms or problems are identified, they can be altered, shifted, and interrupted. At that point, they no longer operate "automatically." At that point, the person beset by the symptom/problem finally experiences himself or herself as a *creator* rather than as a victim of subjective experiences beyond his or her control.

Identities as Trance States: A Teaser

The formation of hypnotic identities is discussed in detail in Chapters 10 and 19. The concept of identity as a trance state is a crucial one when working with Deep Trance Phenomena. In a sense, hypnotic identities are the *"piece de resistance,"* the grand culmination of trance states, which is why they are discussed later in far greater length than this introductory chapter allows. In a nutshell, to be in a trance identity means that we have fused or become one with a set of experiences that defines how we view ourselves. Whether that identity is "I am a loser" or "I am a competent editor," in both cases one's experience of self is *narrowed and circumscribed*. Working with hypnotic identities is one of the most fascinating facets of deep trance therapy.

2

Home Is Where the Trance Is

TRANCES are often a necessary means of surviving and negotiating the physical universe. They are like tunnels you walk through in order to maneuver and focus in the world. Some trances are functional and pleasing; others are dysfunctional and pathological. Some trances will be in alignment with your goals, while others will impede you.

Deep Trance Phenomena are, at one and the same time, a means of survival for the overwhelmed child and the core of symptom structure for the coping adult. Those trance phenomena that create adult symptomatology usually have their origins in childhood patterns of experience.

Erickson (1952/1980) has noted that ". . .hypnosis depends upon inter- and intrapersonal relationships [that] are inconstant and alter in accord with personality reactions to each hypnotic development" (p. 139). The context of Erickson's statement is the induction of therapeutic trance in the therapy session. I have found that patients' abilities to go into therapeutic trance in session stem from a more primary experience of trance as a process of "inter- and intrapersonal relation-ships [that] are inconstant and alter in accord with personality reactions." This more primary experience of trance occurs throughout childhood and forms the basis for the creation and maintenance of Deep Trance Phenomena throughout adulthood. In adulthood, trance as symptom is an *intra*personal (self-to-self) process which was originally generated by a series of *inter*personal (self-to-other) interactions (more on this in Chapter 7).

Each Deep Trance Phenomenon is designed to maintain, support, and protect the integrity of the child. During the early stages of its development, the Deep Trance Phenomenon is *context-dependent*: that is, the particular trance arises in response to a particular stimulus — such as angry remonstrations from Daddy. Gradually, as the usefulness of this Deep Trance Phenomenon increases, it gains a kind of intrapsychic autonomy and is generalized to a wide variety of associated stimuli. In the case of the child who is repeatedly remon-strated by the father, soon all (or most) men who are in positions of authority will evoke the Deep Trance Phenomenon.

Each Deep Trance Phenomenon represents a particular facet or expression of consciousness. Children will create whichever trance states are most helpful in buffering them against the first experience they are not able to integrate. (This type of experience is often labeled as "trauma" or "crisis," but it is really *any* event or inter-action that exceeds the child's capacity to fully feel, process, and integrate.) Each child will have a proclivity toward certain trance states more than others — which is why adults vary so dramatically in their ability to experience the various hypnotic phenomena. *Most adults have had a lifetime of experience in creating the kind of trance states that are most effective in handling their particular circumstances.*

Since the Deep Trance Phenomenon worked so well in its original context, the child then uses it to create an automatic response to the environment *in general*. The environment is no longer experienced *as it is* in the present moment but rather *as it was* in the past. As an adult, the individual brings his past, historical context of family experience with him into the present *via* the creation of one or more Deep Trance Phenomenon. It is therefore the Deep Trance Phenomenon, originally created as a means of protecting the child, that is currently preventing the adult from being *present* in *present time* (more about this point later). Indeed, Erickson noted this characteristic as being indicative of a somnambulistic trance in his 1967 paper, "Further Experimental Investigation of Hypnosis: Hypnotic and Nonhypnotic Realities":

> As a measure of recognizing somnambulistic hypnotic behavior there was a systematic appraisal by the group of the various manifestations that were likely to occur in the behavior of such subjects. . . .These criteria were: . . . .*An apparent inability to perceive external stimuli included in the immediate situation, and the frequent spontaneous ability to misperceive the surrounding realities as the realities experienced or imagined possible in the past of the individual subject, often with peculiar restrictions or alterations in the actual perception of reality.* (p. 29) [Italics added]

Trance states that are created as symptoms appear to possess an autonomy that perpetuates the symptoms. Removing the autonomy of the trance functioning helps to shift the symptom complex. Then, instead of being locked into a rigid stimulus-response pattern, the person has the option of many different responses to the one stimulus. Now there is a variability among trance states. Even if all of those different responses involve trance states, they are trance states the person *chooses* to experience.

Emphasizing Process Over Content

As I mentioned, I presuppose that anyone who is in the grip of a complaint, problem, or a symptom has hypnotized himself or herself into a particular state of consciousness in response to some kind of experience which could not be processed at that moment. Discovering the *content* of the problematic experience is not emphasized in the treatment approaches I describe in this book, however. What is emphasized is *the trance process by which the person ultimately creates the symptom.*

This trance process, which functions "on automatic" in the adult's life, almost always can be traced back to childhood experiences of acute or chronic trauma. Recovering, reliving, even remembering that trauma is not necessary; in fact, I only focus on it when the patient insists on a content connection. My first choice is to move directly into the process of the current symptomatology. If we look at an example of childhood molestation in slow motion, so to speak, and then look at the adult's symptomatology and how to work with it, this difference will become apparent.

A young girl is being molested by her father for the first time. While that action is taking place she creates the responses of, "I'm scared, I'm afraid, I'm bad, it hurts, I can't stand this" — which later function as posthypnotic suggestions in the form of internal dialogues. This is followed by her unconscious creation of one or more Deep Trance Phenomenon to help her escape the experience and her own responses to it. She may develop amnesia ("It never happened"), and/or analgesia ("My body feels fine"), and/or dissociation ("It wasn't so bad"), and/or negative visual hallucination (not seeing her external environment during the trauma), and/or negative auditory hallucination (not hearing the sounds occurring during the trauma), and so forth. At some point, whichever trance states are most successful in helping her survive the ordeal will begin to function automatically.

Twenty years later she arrives for a session with a psychotherapist, complaining that she is non-orgasmic. (Some clients directly express to the therapist, "I want to work on a molest issue involving my father." Others will say, "I'm in a relationship with someone important right now and I can't have an orgasm.") What process is she using to shut down her body's natural sexual response the moment she is in an intimate situation? By asking her to recreate her body sensations as she shuts down, I can begin to identify the trance phenomena involved. *Whether or not you as the therapist discover the content of the trauma that underlies the current symptomatology, you can discover and alter the trance phenomena that create it again and again in present time.* You take the presenting problem — "I can't have an orgasm" — and you let the client show you which Deep Trance Phenomena she uses to create that symptomatic trance.

Most forms of therapy assume that dealing with content is at least *somewhat* necessary for healing. If the client could just get to the first time a certain trauma happened — and either draw it, relive it, dream about it, understand it, analyze it, scream it, symbolize it in imagery, or have its muscular counterparts kneaded — then somehow the effects of the trauma would disappear. By working with the non-experienced event and how it impacted you *then*, somehow it will no longer impact you *now*.

I am suggesting that content — the events that pepper our lives — is secondary. What we create *in response to those events* is primary and constitutes our process. Content is the manifestation of process; our behavior, which is our "content," is the one tangible thing we see in regard to our problems and pathologies. However, the content of our lives — the way we manifest our own internal psychodynamic processes — is a constantly shifting series of events that changes over time. Only the process by which the state-of-being is created threads throughout a common denominator.

Take the example of an adult who complains of agoraphobic reactions. In terms of content, her series of relevant events runs as follows: At the age of three she had an experience with her mother in which she was left alone without a babysitter for several hours. At the age of five, she was not picked up from kindergarten after school one day and got lost as she tried to wander home. At age seven, she was taunted by a group of girls at recess. At ten, at 15, at 22 — experiences and events are continually happening, the content of which is always changing. However, *the process by which the child/adult responds to and integrates those experiences usually has a surprisingly repetitive quality to it*. By focusing on the trance process that underlies the current symptomatology, the trap of revolving content issues is avoided *while the mechanism that sustains them is effectively altered*.

A client comes for therapy about her relationship with "Dan." She starts talking about the specific content of her issues with Dan. This content is certainly different than the content of her problem in previous relationships — it has different twists and turns, whistles and bangles. What is not different is the process by which she created her own experience yet again — her own continuing saga.

If we work with her current content with Dan, we won't be handling the content with her five previous partners, because we won't be touching on the underlying process. To handle one process is to handle all the processes (usually) that have characterized her failed relationships. If she changes the inner and interactional pattern of response that she experienced with Dan, she cannot arrive at the same failed outcome in her next relationship. Why? Because the *process* will have been changed; the "mold" into which she pours her responses and behavior will be an entirely different shape and texture.

All of us have to come to terms with our own content. Most of us have to keep going back and back and back for it, looking for "the answer" in our stories. And while we do get answers — we do piece together the incredible mosaic of cause-and-effect — we often still do not actually feel *better*. Eventually, a turning point comes and we begin to ask, "Where am I now? How can I change the way I experience life *now*?" Feeling *current* restores one's sense of personal power and enhances one's ability to take responsibility for the ongoing moments of experience.

There is a common myth that Erickson disregarded content for process; that clients often found themselves changing without knowing how or why. They had quit smoking or overeating but could not "put their finger on" just what had changed. Certainly, no deep content issues had been addressed —at least none that they could recall.

Actually, Erickson would focus on either process or content, depending on his clinical judgement of each particular case. For example, in one lengthy case cited in *Hypnotherapy: An Exploratory Casebook* (Erickson & Rossi, 1979), Erickson focused on content and insight as an important part of the process of resolving the patient's symptoms:

> Recognizing that a great deal of insight therapy needs to be done in this session, Erickson begins by giving her some "mental warm-up exercises": He requests that she recall in exact detail the furniture of the place she slept the night before and than all the things she saw on a shopping tour yesterday. All of this may seem irrelevant to the patient, but Erickson is thereby "warming up" search operations in her mind with non-threatening material. These search operations will be used later in the session, when she will need to seek and express insights. (p. 207)

In the subsequent paragraph Rossi summarizes Erickson's approach in this session by stating that he "touches on" one of her "basic unconscious complexes" and "then embarks on the work of undoing repressions in a variety of ways. . . . Here we witness Erickson at his best as a therapist facilitating the process of insight....After a great deal of initial resistance, X experiences a flood of insights about her family dynamics and the reasons for her symptoms."

While some of Erickson's therapeutic interventions were aimed at facilitating conscious insight, he is most noted for leaving matters to "autonomous unconscious change." The point is that even when Erickson was focusing on evoking *unconscious* change, content issues were still involved: he meant that the necessary insights and understandings could be grasped on an *unconscious level.* So he was still concerning himself with content to some extent; *what varied was the level of consciousness at which the content was apprehended.*

In discussing the two kinds of therapeutic work, conscious and unconscious, Erickson and Rossi (1979) explain that, first, the patient is introduced to the "difference between the conscious and unconscious mind." Once that is achieved, Erickson will continue to explore on both levels, leaving change on an unconscious level if the patient is willing, or bringing it into conscious awareness if that seems more beneficial:

> The activated. . .associations may remain at an unconscious level, where during trance they are turned over to effect an apparently autonomous resolution of the patient's problem. It is possible that hypnotherapy can take place entirely at an unconscious level without the patient (and sometimes even the therapist) knowing the "why" of the cure. The patient only knows a problem has been resolved. No insight in the conventional analytic sense is involved [because the insight remains unconscious].
>
> . . . .A period of therapeutic trance. . .may [also] stimulate associations to a problem that the patient wants to talk about. This route naturally leads to insight therapy. After an initial experience of trance, the therapist may simply wait for the patient to bring up relevant associations. If none are forthcoming, the therapist may again review the nature and possible sources of the problem to ascertain if the patient now has more access to relevant associations. (p. 165)

Erickson developed many ingenious ways of working with content, one of the most famous of which was his "jigsaw" method of splitting apart the emotional and intellectual aspects of a past trauma (see Appendix III). In the following quotation he describes how he worked with a medical student who was in danger of flunking out of school because he irrationally refused to attend any classes on dermatology. Erickson offered to work with him in front of his classmates, requesting that he first spend the next week "trying to remember what he had forgotten." In summarizing his jigsaw approach, Erickson explains (Erickson & Rossi, 1981):

> Hypnosis can also allow you to divide up your patient's problems. For example, a patient comes to you with some traumatic experience in the past which has resulted in a phobic reaction or an anxiety state. One can put him in a deep trance and suggest that he recover only the emotional aspects of that experience. . . .In other words, one can split off the intellectual aspects of a problem for a patient and leave only the emotional aspects to be dealt with. One can have a patient cry out very thoroughly over the emotional aspects of a traumatic experience and then later let him recover it in a jigsaw fashion — that is, let him recover a little bit of the intellectual content of the traumatic experience of the past, then a little bit of the emotional content — and these different aspects need not necessarily be connected. Thus, you let the young medical student see the pitchfork, then you let him feel the pain he experiences in the gluteal region, then you let him see the color green, then you let him feel himself stiff and rigid, and then you let him feel the full horror of his stiffness and rigidity. *Various bits of the incident recovered in this jigsaw fashion allow you to eventually recover an entire, forgotten traumatic experience of childhood that had been governing this person's behavior in medical school and handicapping his life very seriously.* (pp. 6-7) [Italics added]

Here we see Erickson using therapeutic trance states to "divide up" the patient's traumatic responses (content), which are seen as responsible for his current phobic reaction. A trance is induced and the patient is lead through a carefully orchestrated "jigsaw" experience in which he alternately relives intellectual and emotional aspects of the originating trauma. This is certainly one way of approaching the presenting problem of the student's aversion to the dermatology classes.

Another perhaps simpler and easier way is to simply observe and utilize the trance state underlying the student's current symptomatology. What trance states does he use to create his strong, phobic response? Probably a combination of age regression, pseudo-orientation in time, and negative visual hallucinations. By working solely with these trance phenomena, the phobic reaction can be dissipated, whether or not the original trauma is recovered. Why? Because the current symptomatology cannot be produced without the trance phenomena that comprise it. The Deep Trance Phenomena are the "ingredients" of the phobic "cake."

This brings us to the basic if subtle difference between Erickson's trance approaches and those presented herein. Erickson preferred to use therapeutic trance to work toward "unconscious change" in patients. I prefer to use the symptomatic trance state the patient brings to the session and work toward a "no-trance" state of expanded awareness (more on the "no-trance" state in Chapter 4).

Erickson was also quite willing to work with content, but he would find ingenious ways of doing it (such as dissociating the intellectual and emotional components of a trauma; or using two-level communication to talk directly to the unconscious and evoke inherent resources and abilities; or to reframe the symptom via stories, metaphors, puns, analogies.) In terms of working with process, he would work with the behaviors going on in the moment and utilize them for cues as to how to proceed to evoke resources and new associations.

Erickson's way of working with process was summarized by Rossi (Erickson, Rossi & Rossi, 1976):

> On careful reflection it will be found that this orientation to *process* is more frequently prominent in Erickson's approach than his concern about *content*. In inducing trance, for example, he utilizes the *process* of confusion to depotentiate consciousness; the actual subject matter or content of the confusion is irrelevant. In training a hypnotic subject it is the

process of experiencing one and then a series of hypnotic phenomena that is important, not the content of the particular phenomena. . . .Content, to be sure, is important, but its importance is usually as a vehicle to gain entry to the patient's attention and associative structures where the process of therapy can be facilitated. (p. 224)

This is still different from the type of process work I am describing wherein the person is not "trained" in experiencing various hypnotic phenomena, but rather brings his/her own trance symptoms into the session. Content is used only as a stimulus to help the client recreate the symptom via its underlying Deep Trance Phenomena. Furthermore, my focus is not on evoking resources and associations but on *removing* the barrier of the symptomatic trance state. Once the trance phenomena underlying the problem is shifted, interrupted, reassociated, or dissolved, the person's resources will automatically "float" to the surface.

The next chapter provides introductory case samples of how Deep Trance Phenomena can be worked with in the therapy session.

3

"You Are the Tenth One":
Working With the Self
Behind the Trance

Most of us automatically (or "unconsciously") recreate states of consciousness from the past as trance phenomena in the present. Many states of awareness involve some combination of Deep Trance Phenomenon; any state that is problematic can be assumed to contain one or more trance phenomena. The task of the psychotherapist therefore becomes one of *de-hypnotizing* the client: "awakening" the client's awareness to the deep trance that is being recreated from the original family context and which continues to function, unnoticed, as the invisible "glue" of the client's current-day symptom complex.

In essence, this awakening amounts to *counting* one's *self* in the therapy. Most forms of psychotherapy do not really count the person as a creative self; she is viewed as a product of all the other factors that are counted: her feelings, her thoughts, her associations,

29

her problems, her body sensations, her muscle tonus, her memories, and her dreams. But these are all only *creations* of the self behind the trance, not the person herself, and while this can seem like unnecessary philosophizing, the shift in attitude toward seeing the client as a creative being is a major one.

There is a well-known story from the *Upanishads* that beautifully makes this point about forgetting to count the self. According to the story, there are ten men walking through the woods. They come upon a river, which they must cross. Because the current is so strong, they are afraid that some of them might be washed away, so they decide to hold hands and lock arms as they cross. This way, no one will get lost. They reach the other side and, just to be sure, they decide to count to verify that everyone has made it across.

The first man counts 1, 2, 3, 4, 5, 6, 7, 8, 9. "Somebody is missing!" he shouts in alarm. The next person in line begins to count: 1, 2, 3, 4, 5, 6, 7, 8, 9! "Oh, no! Somebody *is* missing! Who did we lose?" Each person, in turn, counts the lot of them and comes up with only 9 people.

Finally, a sage comes by and, hearing the nature of their complaint, realizes their mistake. He counts them, one by one, and reaches 10. "You are the tenth one," the sage says to each.

How does this story translate in the therapy session? For me it means that the therapist learns to communicate with the creative being, the "self," behind the trance; it is the self that can change the trance and hence the symptom. The reason therapy succeeds or fails is not always due to the skill of the therapist, or to the severity or tenacity of early traumas; nor is it always due to the trance states themselves. It can be due to the being as a creative self.

As I have said, it is my view that whenever a client presents a problem or symptom to me, he or she is also presenting a trance state. Symptom structures are supported by Deep Trance Phenomenon that come in clusters and form an internal latticing of associations and responses that the person experiences as problematic. These clusters of trance phenomena will reveal themselves in an autonomous fashion to the observant therapist.

I mentioned the alcoholic client who, as the session unfolded, spontaneously began to age regress. I requested that she maintain continued eye contact with me during the regression. Quite suddenly she was unable to see me at all (she had negatively hallucinated). The initiating Deep Trance Phenomenon of age regression was now "joined" by that of negative hallucination. These two trance experiences had combined in the client to produce her own unique phenomenology and symptomatology. In my breakthrough moment, I realized that in order for her to create the distance that she had needed to survive as a child, she had to *not see* much of her immediate external environment. It now became clear that the very same dynamics were being used to create the behavior of excessive drinking: she would create trance states in which she age regressed (moved from a self-to-other trance of adult interaction into the self-to-self trance of the hurt child) and then, essentially, she would stop seeing her external environment.

In order for this person to drink excessively, she must first break off any significant interpersonal contact. She must move from an *interpersonal world* in which the self relates to others in the environment (self-to-other trance) to an *intrapersonal world* (self-to-self trance) in which she does not perceive her surroundings. In essence, this drinker must become "lost" or entranced in her own inner world. Any of the Deep Trance Phenomena discussed in this book can be used to achieve the symptomatic shift into self-to-self trance. In this particular case, the Deep Trance Phenomena of age regression and negative hallucination were used by the client to create her behavior of excessive drinking.

Treatment

A symptom can be thought of as the *non-utilization of unconscious resources*. When we are in a symptom state, we are not making use of inner resources that are normally available to us. This happens because the central characteristic of any trance state used to create the symptom is that it *shrinks our focus of attention*. Interestingly, Erickson viewed this as desirable: trance *helped* the person to narrow his focus of attention and become unaware of all extraneous stimuli and concerns. He then made use of this attentional constriction to heighten and consolidate the person's concentration on the problem at hand and to evoke unconscious resources.

Here, this can be seen as a paradox: the person has created a problem, which requires a shrinking of the focus of attention. At the same time, Erickson has the client shrink his or her focus of attention even more, in order to create a therapeutic trance state.

I am suggesting that the reverse is also true: It is this very narrowing or shrinking of attention, *as it functions in the symptomatic trance state*, that locks the person into an automatic response pattern resulting in a non-utilization of unconscious resources.

For example, in the symptomatic trance state of an anxiety attack (*pseudo-orientation in time*), I shrink my focus of attention to such an extent that I feel totally cut off from the world (I move from an interpersonal trance to an intrapersonal trance). I have no idea how the make the attack stop, and that sense of helplessness (*age regression*) escalates the anxiety and even further shrinks my ability to focus on anything but anxiety. I "don't see" the phone (*negative hallucination*) and I "forget" (*amnesia*) that I can pick it up and call a friend; I "forget" that I have had many periods of time that were completely free of anxiety attacks; I "forget" that I have had control over countless past situations in my life. All of these resources remain untapped by me as long as my intense self-to-self trance—with its shrunken focus of attention and the Deep Trance Phenomena of pseudo-orientation in time and amnesia—remains in tact. In this state I imagine a very vivid and frightening future that is devoid of options and solutions and filled with the uncontrollable, assaultive sensations of anxiety attacks.

Any interruption, shift, or alteration of the Deep Trance Phenomena that is creating the anxiety attack, however, will provide access to the otherwise non-utilized resources. The resources can now "float" to the surface of consciousness. I suddenly remember that a day ago I felt fine, I now can see the phone on my desk, and I think of calling my friend to talk about it. In short, I have "popped out" of my identification with the Deep Trance Phenomena creating the anxiety attack, and once "outside," resources become readily available. In everyday life, any appropriate stimulus can interrupt or alter the Deep Trance Phenomenon: my phone might ring, I remember an important call I need to make, I discover I am out of toilet paper and have to go to the market!

In the therapy setting, the therapist can directly facilitate an interruption, shift, or alteration of the symptomatic trance state. In the case of the alcoholic woman described above, I began to differentiate various aspects of her experience of fogging me out of her vision (her *negative hallucination*) by suggesting slight variations in the fog she was seeing. Was the fog transparent? Opaque? Translucent? Did it have any colors in it? Did it have any texture? In answering my questions, she thereby made differentiations in what had been an undifferentiated mass.

Once she could no longer follow the path of her customary negative hallucination that created her symptom of excessive drinking, she was gradually able to stop. All in all, her treatment spanned six months of intensive work. Although many kinds of treatment interventions were used in working with her symptom of alcoholism, the critical one was interrupting and altering the deep trance patterns of negative hallucination and age regression.

I should mention that I require clients who are drug- and alcohol-addicted to participate in some twelve-step program while they are also working in therapy. Attending these groups helps to remove denial (*amnesia*), to create additional awareness of the addictive issues, and, of course, provide a network of support.

By asking clients to describe their symptoms *while breathing and looking at me*, I interrupt the self-to-self trance of the symptom by placing them (via eye contact) in a self-to-other trance with me. This changes the context in which the symptom occurs and adds the therapist as a resource in present time. (This is a common technique in Gestalt therapy and was demonstrated to me in 1975 by Eric Marcus, M.D., and Jack Rosenberg, Ph.D.) Erickson has pointed out that the adult in present time has resources that the traumatized child did not have. By keeping the client focused in the present, she is able to take the present with her into the past. This differs from therapies which have the adult re-experience past traumas without the buffer of present-time resources. Therapists need to understand that the client survived the trauma and later created resources to cope with it. To pretend those resources are not currently present and that the client needs to relive the trauma without them, is to needlessly dramatize a situation again that no longer reflects the present.

As an example, let's take the young woman above who complains of being non-orgasmic. I might say:

"Jill, when you are having sex, at the moment that you go numb or space out or freeze up, I would like you to get a three-dimensional picture of the moment you freeze up. You might see this picture in your mind's eye, or perhaps floating in front of us in the room. Notice your muscles. . .Tell me which are tight and which are loose . . .Notice what you are saying to yourself. . .What kinds of thoughts are going through your mind?"

While recreating her symptom-trance, Jill might answer slowly: "My shoulders are tight. . .my jaw is tight. . .my stomach is tight. . .I'm holding my breath. . .I'm thinking to myself, *Don't touch me, don't come near me, don't hurt me.*"

"All right, Jill, what I'd like you to do is to merge with that picture. . .Continue to hold your muscles tightly *while you breathe and look at me.*"

> In order for a symptom to remain a symptom, there has to be a holding of the breath. This holding allows the person to shift into a self-to-self trance: he or she is no longer present with you but is back watching an old internal movie and re-experiencing a past event (*age regression*). When I request that clients continue to experience the symptom while they breathe and look at me, I am offering them the possibility of experiencing their symptoms fully *but with me in present time.* This initial directive ("breathe and look at me") *now includes the world in what previously was a very fixed trance* and lays the groundwork for the therapeutic variations in the trance that are suggested later.

> Requesting the direct, sustained eye contact further helps to stimulate or trigger those clusters of Deep Trance Phenomena that already function autonomously within clients as defense mechanisms that help shield them from the intensity of interpersonal contact.

After a few minutes I observe a change in the intensity of Jill's eye contact and ask, "What's going on right now?"

"I guess I'm just spacing out." [*Dissociation*]

"What I'd like you to do is space out even more *while you breathe and look at me.*"

> At this point I recognize that she is beginning to demonstrate for me the process of how she goes about *not* having an

orgasm: "I tighten my shoulder muscles, I tighten my jaw, I tighten my stomach, and I space out." It is likely that this is the process she created to handle her early molest trauma.

I repeat, "Now breathe and look at me."

"I can't see you very clearly. . .you seem foggy to me."

"Foggy? And as your vision continues to get foggier and foggier, *breathe and look at me.*"

She continues to teach me how she does the trance of "no orgasm" through her use of Deep Trance Phenomena:

—she goes numb by tightening her muscles [*sensory distortion*]
—she "spaces out" [*dissociation*]
—she fogs her vision [*negative hallucination*].

All the lines of early defense pop up in the form of these Deep Trance Phenomena.

At this point the client is experiencing what I call a "fixed trance"; it has no variability. It functions autonomously and it is *context-independent*: she carries it with her into all her relationships and life experiences. If I as a clinician can offer her variations to her characteristic Deep Trance Phenomena, then I am beginning the process of *altering the symptom by interrupting the Deep Trance Phenomena that hold the symptom structure together*. In our above case, I begin to interrupt the established stimulus-response pattern of her tightening her muscles in response to the physical presence of a man by suggesting a vast array of variations around one or more of her Deep Trance Phenomenon. For example:

"Now as you breathe and look at me, you might notice that part of the fog is thinner, and part of it is moving, and another part of it is thick and dense."

Another is to utilize her own posthypnotic suggestions (*"Don't touch me, don't come near me, don't hurt me"*) in a way that creates a healing communication (see Chapter 10).

All these differentiations to the undifferentiated mass of the fog create a varying experience in what was a *fixed trance state*. They also help to create a parallel state of consciousness (the "witness" or objective observer, to be discussed later) that can interact with the autonomous Deep Trance Phenomenon and thereby alter it. As each

Deep Trance Phenomenon is differentiated via alternative associations, the symptoms which are created by the fixed trance lose their vehicle of manifestation.

Another example that involves anorexia-bulimia may further amplify these points. Several Deep Trance Phenomena are usually involved in creating this disorder. *Positive hallucinations* allow the person to perceive a large-sized body where, in reality, there is a very thin body; meanwhile, *posthypnotic suggestions* (usually internalized parental messages) sustain the internal cognitions that help to distort the person's visual perceptions; *age regression* keeps the person at the emotional level when the initial trance phenomena were created for purposes of survival.

When I began working with a woman whose presenting complaint was anorexia-bulimia, I had no idea what Deep Trance Phenomena were creating her behavior. My attitude was one of intense curiosity. "I'm fascinated. Teach me how you create anorexia-bulimia. When you are on the verge of bingeing on the 10 bags of potato chips you eat a day, what does your body feel like? Can you describe the sensations you feel? Can you make a picture of that intense moment when you are beginning to want to binge? *As you breathe and look at me*, recreate that moment. . .*As you breathe and look at me*, just let yourself recreate that moment. . ."

As she begins to duplicate her past trance state, she slips into a trance that deepens quite rapidly. She shifts her body position in the chair, draws her feet up toward her chest and curves her arms around her legs, intertwining them in a tight grip.

I say softly, "Just continue to *breathe and look at me. Breathe and look at me*. . .What are your thoughts. . .What are your sensations?"

She answers in a muffled, faraway voice, "Don't be close to me. . . don't touch me. . . don't come near me."

As I sit and observe her, this woman is showing me how she goes into trance to create her symptomatology. Interestingly, there is little to no self-consciousness involved in this particular approach, because the very focus on habitual trances assures clients that they will be protected. On the other hand, if I had said, "Let's begin to handle your molest issue," resistances would rebound. When I asked my client to demonstrate for me how she "did" anorexia-bulimia, I was asking her *to go into the trance she was already in.*

When I realized she was verbalizing for me the posthypnotic suggestions she had placed on automatic to protect her from future molests, I saw my task as one of creating a variability in her fixed trance state. I used the exact words she had already given me, but I spoke them in a very specific way by splitting apart the positive and negative injunctions in the sentences.

Looking into her left eye I said softly, almost inaudibly, "Don't." Now shifting to look directly into her right eye, I said more emphatically, *"Be close to me."*

Don't	Be close to me
Don't	Touch me
Don't	Come near me

With the use of carefully modulated vocal cues and eye contact, I have shifted the trance by shifting the emphasis on the posthypnotic suggestions. This allows a new message to become available—a message that contains suggestions for her to begin utilizing those specific unconscious and non-utilized resources that are intimately connected with her problem area. While the conscious mind may be hearing the old message, "Don't be close to me," the unconscious mind hears the new resource, *"Be close to me,"* that was previously unavailable. (See also Chapter 10 on Posthypnotic Suggestion.)

Here again I have observed the client and identified the Deep Trance Phenomena that she presented; and I have altered her fixed trance state by differentiating the posthypnotic suggestions that comprised it.

Each major Deep Trance Phenomenon will be explored in terms of how it manifests in various adult symptomatology and how it can be altered therapeutically. In the next chapter, we will examine the important theoretical, therapeutic, and experiential reasons for making a distinction between states of trance, no-trance, and therapeutic trance.

4

Trance Or No-Trance? Marrying East and West

As I MENTIONED in Chapter 1, what I call the "no-trance state," Ericksonian hypnotherapists call "therapeutic trance," and the Eastern meditative traditions call "meditation." We are all looking at a similar phenomenon—our most natural and optimal state-of-being—but through different lenses. In Asia water is called *paune*, in Europe it is called *aqua*, in the Middle East it is called *mai*. It's the same substance, whatever you call it. In an analogous manner the *natural state*, the *no-trance state*, the *therapeutic trance state*, and the *meditative state* are all different words describing a similar phenomenological experience. This natural state has no boundaries that separate the individual from the rest of the cosmos. Pain and problems arise only when we leave this state and identify ourselves with limiting ideas.

Because meditation is often misunderstood in the West, its relation to hypnotherapy is also likely to be misunderstood. Briefly, let us compare the two.

Meditation is often discussed in terms of three stages: *darana*, which is the practice of concentrating on a fixed point; *dhyana*, which is the point at which the focus of attention becomes an unbroken flow of concentration; and *samadhi*, which is a total cessation of the subject-object relationship. Samadhi occurs when the boundaries between the person who is concentrating and the object being concentrated upon disappear. As *samadhi* continues, dispassion follows; the individual loses all tendencies to become identified with the contents of the mind.

This is similar to being in a therapeutic trance wherein there is a free flow of associations without identification, attachment, or interruption. Thoughts, feelings, and emotions pass through the person without the ordinary damper of judgments or labels. In meditation, this experience occurs as the meditator witnesses the flow of mental contents without attaching to them.

To superimpose these terms on a Western framework, Erickson's hypnotherapeutic techniques constitute *dharna*, the means by which a person's attention was focused and narrowed, allowing the person to then slip into "therapeutic trance"—or *dhyana meditation*. What differentiates therapeutic trance from meditation is that in therapeutic trance, the mind and its contents are worked with—they are reframed, reassociated, utilized, reinterpreted, dissociated, and so on. In meditation the mind is simply observed without intervention. In therapeutic trance, a problem is being presented for change. In meditation, the only problem is one's identification with one's thoughts and experiences.

Along those same lines of thinking, the natural state, or the no-trance state, or the therapeutic trance state is a *no-position position*. Erickson reported an experience that well describes this notion of a no-position position. In an interview with Ernest Rossi, he talked about his encounter with "*the middle of nowhere*" (Erickson & Rossi, 1977/1980):

> E: I was in the backyard a year ago in the summertime. I was wondering what far-out experience I'd like to have. As I puzzled over that, I noticed that I was sitting out in the middle of nowhere....I was just an object in space. Of all the buildings I couldn't see an outline. I couldn't see the chair in which I was sitting; in fact, I couldn't feel it....*I was just an object and all alone with me was an empty void. No buildings, earth, stars,*

sun. . . .It was one of the most pleasing experiences. What is this? Tremendous comfort. . . . Inside the stars, the planets, the beaches. I couldn't feel the weight. (pp. 129-130) [Italics added]

In what I am calling the no-trance state (also in *samadhi* and *satori*) there is a clear sense of non-identification (yogis call this "dispassion"); there is a sense of flow, a sense of perceptions coming and going, a sense of being and perceiving without judgment or identification. Erickson called his taste of this experience "being in the middle of nowhere." By contrast, in trance states of identification we constrict our focus of attention and fuse with each and every occurrence in the day; our sense of self and well-being fluctuate commensurately.

One of my clients put it this way:

I am very familiar with that feeling of coming and going. It's a feeling of things *passing through* me and I can see them all. Nothing sticks, nothings gets interrupted in its flow. It's a very rich, very free space to be in. I feel at my best in that state—especially when I can carry it into work situations. At my job, large volumes of things pass through me—people's requests and demands, personnel dynamics, political considerations, and so forth.

I have trouble when it feels like all these elements come and hit something solid—that would be your trance state. When the outer flow hits something solid in me, I begin to lose my good feeling and feel myself shrink down and contract (trance). Then I get confused, disoriented and even a little bit dissociated. I can't keep track of things, I can't process the flow anymore. Everything sticks, stops, and halts. I literally have to stop and go outside, or go into a vacant room and just "space out" for a few minutes. I let myself veer back into that expanded space and then I feel better. I feel like I can cope again.

The trance states we normally call *feelings* ("I feel good," "I feel bad," "I am being rejected") are the states in which attention is shrunken and focused, identified and attached. These are the states that breed symptomatology. This is what patients bring to you.

The Ericksonian concept of therapeutic trance is phenomeno-logically quite similar to the Eastern concept of meditation and *samadhi*. In that framework, this state of being is not a trance state at all; rather, it is the transcendence of limiting states of mind and being. I find it fascinating that some of the best descriptions of therapeutic trance in Ericksonian literature beautifully express what I now call the *no-trance* state of Eastern meditative traditions. For example, Gilligan writes (1987):

> . . .in trance I can feel both "here" and "there," connected with you and disconnected from you, "a part of" and "apart from" an experience. This. . . gives rise to a nonconceptual and nonverbal experiential state of unity. It is a more primary, inclusive way of relating than the separating, "either/or" logic characterizing analytical, conscious process. In other words, *trance processes tend to unify relations* ("this" and "that"), while *conscious processes tend to differentiate relations* ("this" *vs.* "that"). . . .[These features of trance] suggest trance as a state of deep experiential absorption where a person can operate independently from the constraints of regulatory, error-oriented conscious process. (p. 42)

Two more passages by Gilligan (1987):

> The hypnotized subject usually feels little need to *try* to do anything or the compulsion to "plan ahead." Experience "just seems to happen" and "flows quite effortlessly." (p. 43)

> [Trance] can allow a person to disidentify with and move beyond certain attachments (e.g., to pain, a behavior pattern, a perceptual style). . . .Trance is an opportunity to return to a basic essence of one's identity. (p. 43)

The Paradox of It All

In Erickson's therapeutic trance state (which I call no-trance), he takes a patient's symptomatology, focuses it further, and thereby helps the person enter a more natural state in which thoughts, feelings, emotions and associations come and go in a state of deep relaxation and comfort. This is similar to the meditative state prior to *samadhi*.

This brings us to the classic paradoxical truism that the symptom is the cure. In *Gestalt Therapy Now* (1970), editors Fagan and Shepard described what they termed the "law of paradoxical change." Simply put, whatever thought or emotion is completely experienced disappears into something else and the experiencer enters a deepened state of well-being. Erickson had his own understanding and application of paradox: The patient was presented with the paradoxical task of not only further experiencing the symptom but also worsening it. Erickson believed that such an approach demonstrated to the patient his or her ability to change the symptomatology. The implication is, *If you can make it worse in response to my request, you can also make it better.*

In Rossi's application of symptom prescription (Rossi, 1986), he explains its effectiveness in terms of his "state-dependent theory of hypnosis." By asking the patient to experience and worsen the symptom, "we are presumably turning on right-hemispheric processes that have a readier access to the state-dependent encoding of the problem." This means that the therapist is thus working with the actual ingredients (psychobiological states) of the problem, rather than with its rarefied, cognitive version.

The means by which a therapeutic outcome is evoked from a symptomatic state comes through the narrowing and fixating of attention, which eventually triggers a spontaneous *expansion* of attention. A phobia, as it is experienced chronically by a person, requires an intensely shrunken focus of attention. I would treat the phobia by intensifying that experience of narrowed focus and thereby lead the patient into an expanded state of comfort, relaxation, and deep change (therapeutic trance). The symptom itself is used to create a more therapeutic natural state.

It is paradoxical. Intensifying the dynamic that creates the symptomatology actually helps the person move out of it into an expanded state. In other words, the more you shrink your focus of attention in therapeutic trance, the more your perspective spontaneously expands (a no-trance state, in my terms).

Gilligan has noted the paradoxical nature of trance (1987):

"Trance involves a paradoxical, both/and logic. That is, a person identifies with both sides of a complementary distinction of 'this' and 'that,' 'inside' and 'outside,' 'subject' and 'object'" (pp. 40-41).

In the *no-trance* state I am describing, the person becomes larger than or contains both sides of "this" and "that," allowing them to exist. Identification with either side is so reduced that an integration naturally and effortlessly occurs—many times on a nonverbal level. Often, clients experience a deep comprehension of both sides of their issue without identifying with either.

The same principle is true in meditation. As mentioned, in the practice of *dharna* or *dhyana*, one's attention is concentrated on a single point or object. By doing so, "you" (the small you of identifications and attachments) will eventually disappear and "YOU" (the larger you behind all these creations) will enter into your natural state.

Here is the point of intersection between Erickson's therapeutic trance state, my no-trance state, and the Eastern tradition as represented in the philosophy of Tao. In the words of Lao-tzu (1958):

> In order to contract a thing, one should show his standard first; in order to weaken, one will surely strengthen first; in order to overthrow, one will surely exalt first; in order to take, one will surely give first.

This is called "subtle wisdom" in the Tao, and it also reflects what contemporary clinicians call the law of paradoxical change: to change something, increase it rather than trying to undo it. If attention is already shrunken, shrink it *more*; amplify problematic emotional responses rather than trying to make them decrease. By doing this, you will become part of the Tao (according to Eastern wisdom, Tao-te Ching, Chapter 36), you will enter Erickson's state of therapeutic trance, and you will enter what I call the no-trance state. They are all similar, in essence.

The paradox of "symptom as cure" as it relates to Eastern traditions is perhaps best illustrated in the experience of the Zen koan. Rossi and Jichaku describe the paradoxical process by which a Zen student uses the intense focus of the koan to enter an expanded state (Rossi & Ryan, 1991):

The koan is used as a single point of contemplative focus; and single-mindedly, in response to the Roshi's instruction to become intimate or "one" with the koan, the aspirant absorbs himself into a recursive, subvocal inquiry or review of the koan. After some period of such inquiry (it may be years), the moment finally arrives when the aspirant becomes so intimately absorbed, so concentrated in the koan, that *the review of the koan becomes an autonomous and effortless action: the koan breathes the koan,* as when, by comparative analogy, music may "play" the musician during periods of creative inspiration. In the midst of this condition or level of awareness, called *satori* in Zen, there is no consciousness of "I" as a personal construct. All dualistic rational distinctions between self and other, subjective and objective, inner and outer, are totally annihilated [notice the similarity to Erickson's experience described above]. There is only the koan which engages in everyday activities and experiences —the koan laughs and weeps, walks and rests, stands up and sits down.

During this condition—described in the literature as "pure like clear water, like a serene mountain lake, not moved by any wind" (Aitken, 1978)—*the mind is ready and open for a spontaneous realization experience. At this point, any external or internal stimuli can catalyze an abrupt realization experience. It could be the sound of a temple bell, or the sight of peach blossoms in the distance, or an experience of physical pain.*

The Master Hakuin's story dramatically illustrates the importance of single-minded absorption and, subsequently, how any sudden or unexpected attention-fixating stimulus can precipitate Enlightenment. As the story is told, Hakuin was meditating on *Mu*, one of the most basic and popular Zen koans. In the Mu Koan, a monk asks Joshu in all earnestness, "Has a dog the Buddha nature or not?" Joshu said, "Mu" (translated as "No, does not have"). Hakuin (1686-1769) described his experience as follows (Yampolski, 1971):

"Night and day I did not sleep; I forgot both to eat and rest. Suddenly a great doubt [experience of absorption] manifested itself before me. It was as though I were frozen solid in the midst of an ice sheet extending tens of thousands of miles. A purity filled my breast and I could neither go forward nor retreat. To all intents and purposes I was out of my mind and *Mu* [koan] alone remained. Although I sat in the Lecture Hall and listened to the Master's lecture, it was as though I were hearing a discussion from a distance outside the hall. At times it felt as though I was floating through the air.

"This state lasted for several days. Then I chanced to hear the sound of the temple bell and I was suddenly transformed. It was as if a sheet of ice had been smashed or a jade tower had fallen with a crash. Suddenly I returned to my senses. I felt then that I had achieved the status of Yen-t'ou, who through the three periods of time encountered not the slightest loss (although he had been murdered by bandits). All my former doubts vanished as though ice had melted away. In a loud voice I called: 'Wonderful, wonderful. There is no cycle of birth and death through which one must pass. There is no enlightenment one must seek. The seventeen-hundred koans handed down from the past have not the slightest value whatsoever.' " [In press, italics added]

What I call *no-trance*, what Erickson calls "therapeutic trance," and meditation all involve complete absorption in an object—as in the above case, a koan. But it could be a spot on the wall, a crystalline rock, or the request to "breathe and look at me." In meditation a mantra or special object of interest is typically used to promote the experience of shrinking the focus of attention and becoming disidentified or detached. My *no-trance* state and Erickson's therapeutic trance are equivalent to the experience of *not* narrowing one's focus of attention by identifying and attaching. As mentioned, samadhi and other high states of meditation take this experience even further by dissolving the very boundary between subject and object.

Along more mundane lines, any activity that requires you to

shrink your focus of attention for a period of time will eventually give you a "high," "zoned," "expanded" and deeply relaxed feeling. People do needle-point to *relax*. They actually voluntarily choose to shrink their focus of attention down to pinhead scope for hours at a time. Why? Because by doing this incredibly tedious and narrow work, they end up feeling better. Doing needle-point is a kind of meditation in which you shrink your focus of attention to such a degree that you "automatically" pop into an expanded states of awareness.

In the non-pathological trance state of meditation (pre-samadhi), *and* in the pathological trance state that produces symptomatology, *and* in the non-pathological excursions into various "common everyday trances," there is a narrowing of attention. The difference is: In the non-pathological trance states, the narrowing is voluntary and leads to an expanded awareness. I sit down to meditate by choice; I pick up needle point consciously and intentionally. In the symptomatic trance state, the narrowing is involuntary and the trance "pops up" and remains as the dominating characteristic. I stay in that state of shrunken attention *and* I identify with the contents of whatever I'm narrowing my focus of attention down to.

In hypnosis we help clients narrow their attention until they spontaneously (and paradoxically) pop into a more expanded, "therapeutic" state—just like in meditating on koans or doing needle point.

The Wu-wei (1967) states:

An action does not mean doing nothing and keeping silent, but everything be allowed to do what it *naturally* does so that its nature will be satisfied. If one refrains from acting contrary to nature or going against the grain of things, one is in harmony with the tao and thus ones' action will be successful. By non-action, everything can be done, which means going with what is.

This describes the *no-trance* state, since everything is allowed to do what it does.

Aikido, a Japanese art of self-defense, provides a marvelous physical embodiment of the principle of paradoxical change that Erickson demonstrated on the psychotherapeutic level. Note the

obvious points of intersection in the following description of the
main principles of Aikido by Charles Tart (1987):

> The second principle [of Aikido] is to *blend* or harmonize
> with the attack. You practice *Ai.* In the above example of
> being punched, if you had spent months of training,
> strengthening and hardening your abdominal muscles, you
> would be able to defend yourself—not by getting off the
> line but instead by blending and absorbing your attacker's
> punch. . . .To truly harmonize with the attack, you would
> not only get off the line, you also would *not* slow the punch
> down or oppose it in any way. In fact, you might put your
> hand on the punching arm and add energy to it in the
> direction it was already going. You have harmonized and
> blended with the energy of the attack. *By projecting your
> energy in the same direction the attacker projects his, you
> see your attacker's point of view.*
>
> . . . .The third basic principle after you have gotten off the
> line and harmonized with your attacker's energy is to *lead
> that energy further than it originally intended to go, thus
> taking control of it. Then you can throw or otherwise
> control your attacker. The attacker thus provides most of
> the energy for handling his attack.* (pp. 337-338) [Italics
> added]

What an excellent summary of the Ericksonian principle of
utilization, formulated hundreds of years ago in an entirely independent context! When read from the perspective of Aikido
philosophy, the notion of *going with* the direction of the individual's
energy rather than trying to obstruct or divert it does not seem
paradoxical at all—it seems quite logical!

Another way of stating this principle of paradox as it applies to
therapy is, *by asking clients to do what it is they do, trance naturally
occurs.* They shrink their focus of attention, and by doing so, they
pop into a no-trance state —which means they are in a state of
comfort and harmony, free of attachments and identifications.

Meditation contains the same paradox: by narrowing the focus
of attention, the attention eventually becomes diffused and detached.

How does this idea translate into everyday life? We go out into
the world in a no-trance or natural state. Then we lose ourselves (we

get caught up in various trance states) as we focus our attention and marshall our identifications to accomplish various tasks. We make judgments, evaluations, and decisions demanded in our work, and then we identify with each—we fuse with it instead of letting it flow through us. That fusion or state of identification is a trance state— a state of narrowed and contracted focus.

The lived art here is to learn how to take the no-trance state into work situations so that you observe the comings and goings of your own thoughts and feelings without becoming attached to them in a narrowed, fixated trance state. The content of your day rises and subsides in your "space," in your no-trance space. You are the space—you are not your thoughts, feelings and emotions.

Emotion means outward motion. From the perspective of the human potential movement (which includes Gestalt, Reichian, Psychodrama, and all kinds of therapies that focus on the body and emotions), neurosis is caused by an interruption in the outward flow or expression of emotion. If you are in your natural state (my no-trance state), there is no interruption of any motion—of any thought, feeling, sensation or physical movement. What causes interruptions? Our judgments about what we are thinking and feeling, our internal censor who evaluates and identifies with this side of the coin instead of that side of the coin.

The distinction between a trance and a no-trance state is, did you create it or did it just happen to you? In a trance state the experience happens *to* you, which means that you forget the larger Self behind the experience as you shrink your focus of attention to fit into that experience. You are not in touch with the fact that you are the creator of the trance you are experiencing. In a no-trance state, you are aware of yourself as the creator of the experience, which then moves you *beyond* the experience.

5

It's All in the Playing: A Context of Approaches

*P*ERHAPS this is an appropriate time to establish a context for this approach in relation to the field of psychotherapy in general and the Ericksonian model of hypnotherapy in particular.

Erickson introduced the naturalistic/utilization approaches to trance work and therapy that have become the foundation for a paradigmatic shift in the entire field of psychotherapy. In my work with Ericksonian principles, I became convinced that Erickson's naturalistic approaches could be integrated with Eastern orientations and perspectives. The key puzzle pieces—*trance states, interrupting patterns of response*, and *symptoms*—were present in each. The differences between the two approaches arose in how each of these puzzle pieces related to the other.

In the Eastern view, trance states are continually coming and going; the purpose of meditating is to learn to develop some part of the awareness so that it can watch or observe the flow of the trances and the flow of consciousness. This observing part is thereby no longer identified with the ebb and flow of mental life. (In the next chapter, I will discuss how this process of observing or "witnessing" is used to create a therapeutic interpersonal context for change.)

When I moved out of a focus on Eastern orientations and back into Western therapeutic approaches, I found myself drawn to the Deep Trance Phenomena of hypnosis. I had no conscious understanding of why I was so attracted to this particular facet of hypnotic work. I felt compelled to understand what Deep Trance Phenomena were on an experiential level and apart from their circumscribed use in hypnotherapy. What I realized was that *trance states are a crucial part of the fabric of our daily life experience as well as of our symptomatology.*

In the Ericksonian model, I learned that *trance states* could be induced or facilitated as a therapeutic intervention to *interrupt the symptom structure* and *access unconscious potentials and resources.*

In my breakthrough moment, those puzzle pieces came together in an entirely new pattern: I saw that although trance states *can* be used to evoke resources and change on an unconscious level, they can also be—*are used*—to create the symptomatology with which we all struggle. I saw that the person who brings his or her problems and symptoms to me is *already in a trance state*, and that *it is this very trance state that is interrupting his or her experience of the present moment, blocking unconscious potentials and resources, and creating problems and symptoms.* The therapeutic intervention then involves working with the trance state the person has already created (which *de-hypnotizes* him/her), rather than inducing or facilitating another kind of trance that may or may not be pivotal to the patient's symptom structure.

Certainly Erickson viewed trance states as natural occurrences in daily life and even coined the now well-used term, "common everyday trance." Erickson's conception of trance revolutionized the classical view of trance in hypnosis literature as being something that is solely induced or suggested by the operator. Yet Erickson nonetheless regarded trance as something to be induced via the presentation of various indirect (or direct) techniques. For example, in the opening paragraph of his 1952 article entitled "Deep Hypnosis and Its Induction," he writes (Erickson, 1952/1980):

A primary problem in all hypnotic work is the induction of satisfactory trance states. Especially is this true in any work

based upon deep hypnosis. Even the problem of inducing
light trance states and maintaining them at a constant level
is often a difficult task. (p. 139)

. . . .Ordinarily a total of four to eight hours of initial
induction training is sufficient. Then, since trance induction is one process and trance utilization is another—to
permit the subjects to reorganize behavioral processes in
accord with projected hypnotic work, time must necessarily
be allotted with full regard for their capacities to learn and
to respond. (p. 143)

Here trance induction is viewed as a "problem" and a "difficult
task" requiring several hours of skilled work. Since I view anyone
with a problem as being in trance already, I prefer to *observe* and
then *utilize* the trance that is spontaneously presented. This is an
effortless process on the part of the therapist. In my understanding
of Erickson's work, he attempted to create a new trance to counter
the trance the client was already in. I am suggesting that, instead of
creating something *new* in the form of another trance, work with the
trance that is presented. The goal in both approaches is the same: in
Erickson's terms, *therapeutic trance*; in my terms, *no-trance*. Both
refer to that natural state of receptivity in which the self experiences
a sense of intrinsic well-being.

There is a subtle but important difference between utilizing
presenting *behavior* and the presenting *trance*: Erickson observed
and utilized minimal cues of the *presenting behavior* in order to
narrow and fixate attention and induce a trance. I am interested in
observing and utilizing the *presenting Deep Trance Phenomena*
that are creating the symptom. The immediate behavior may be
secondary and derivative in relation to the underlying trance
mechanisms that are *ongoing*. I utilize only what is presented as the
symptomatic trance(s) by having the client re-create it in present
time.

Erickson's utilization approach focused on utilizing presenting
behavior (often in the form of minimal cues) to induce or facilitate
trance experience. He created many ingenious ways of circumventing
the patient's resistances to trance experience by utilizing those very
resistances. In the following excerpt, for example, we see his
creative use of suggestion as a means of redefining *any* response the

patient makes as responsive behavior. A person "who is not receptive to suggestions for hand levitation" can be told a series of
carefully worded suggestions that, in essence, converts what is
normally viewed as non-responsive behavior into responsive behavior (Erickson, 1952/1980):

> One often reads in the literature about subject resistance
> and the techniques employed to circumvent or overcome it.
> In the author's experience the most satisfactory procedure
> is that of accepting and utilizing the resistance as well as
> any other type of behavior, since properly used, they can all
> favor the development of hypnosis. This can be done by
> wording suggestions in such a fashion that a positive or a
> negative response, or an absence of response, are all defined
> as responsive behavior. For example, *a resistive subject
> who is not receptive to suggestions for hand levitation can
> be told*, "Shortly your right hand, or it may be your left
> hand, will begin to lift up, or it may press down, or it may
> not move at all, but we will wait to see just what happens.
> . . .The really important thing is not whether your hand lifts
> up or presses down or just remains still; rather, it is your
> ability to sense fully whatever feelings may develop in your
> hand."
>
> . . . .The subjects whose resistance is manifested by failure
> to hand levitation can be given suggestions that their right
> hand will levitate, their left hand will not. To resist suc-
> cessfully, contrary behavior must be manifested. The result
> is that the subjects find themselves responding to sugges-
> tion, but to their own satisfaction. (p. 154) [Italics added]

I now believe that a person's resistance to one particular type of
trance experience comes from the fact that he or she *is already in
another trance state*. It is unnecessary to circumvent the patient's
resistance to *the trance he is already in* because *that particular trance*
is the substance of his symptomatology.

In the above passage Erickson notes that "the most satisfactory
procedure [for overcoming resistance] is that of accepting and
utilizing the resistance as well as any other type of behavior, since
properly used, they can all favor the development of hypnosis." I

have found that the most satisfactory approach to dealing with resistance is to avoid the possibility of evoking it. I do this by asking the client to *duplicate* or *recreate* the trance state that she is already using to create her symptomatology. Instead of suggesting (either directly or indirectly) a hand levitation, an experience of time distortion, or an amnesia for trance work, I allow the client complete autonomy in producing the trances that are most intrinsic to her states of being. In that way it is the client who selects which trance states he or she will experience. I then merely observe and utilize.

In the above case of the client with anorexia-bulimia, for example, an Ericksonian approach typically might involve giving indirect suggestions for amnesia so that when she went shopping, she would forget to buy the potato chips; or perhaps negative hallucination would have been suggested so that she could pass right by the potato chips without noticing them. Either way, a Deep Trance Phenomenon is being suggested or induced as a way of blocking the occurrence of the symptom or interrupting its pattern of manifestation.

In the approach I am describing, by contrast, the Deep Trance Phenomenon that is already functioning at the core of the person's symptomatology is allowed to manifest to the fullest extent possible, and then *it* is worked with therapeutically. It is that already occurring trance state that is itself creating the symptom and interrupting the person's experience of inner and outer resources available in the present moment.

Once this trance state is taken off "automatic," the symptom structure can begin to dissipate.

Erickson and Rossi believe that "habitual frames of reference" must be depotentiated or bypassed in order to induce/facilitate a therapeutic trance experience (Erickson & Rossi, 1976):

> Erickson believes that the purpose of clinical induction is to focus attention inward and alter some of the ego's habitual patterns of functioning. Because of the limitations of a patient's habitual frames of reference, his usual everyday consciousness cannot cope with certain inner and/or outer realities, and the patient recognizes he has a "problem." Depotentiating a patient's usual everyday conscious sets is thus a way of depotentiating facets of his personal limitations. . . . (p. 448)

By contrast, I believe that the person arrives with his attention already absorbed in and limited by his presenting trance symptomatology. Clusters of Deep Trance Phenomena "hold" the person's attention and constitute what Erickson and Rossi call "limitations of a patient's habitual frames of reference." In their approach, these frames of reference are obstacles that must be bypassed or depotentiated in order to access unconscious processes and resources; in my approach, they are Deep Trance Phenomena that must be utilized and amplified in order to access the no-trance state that permits an uninterrupted flow of both conscious and unconscious processes.

In the next chapter we will explore how the therapist creates *an interpersonal context between him/herself and the client* that allows the client's symptomatic Deep Trance Phenomena to emerge in the therapy session.

6

Creating Context:
You Are Not Your Problem

THE BEGINNING STAGE of therapy for any problem or symptom is helping the person to *disidentify* from the presenting issue. We need to have the new and different experience of discovering that we are *more than* or *larger than* the source of distress with which we are so typically identified.

For example, if I come into therapy with the complaint that "I want intimacy, but I'm afraid to get that close," believing that my fear of intimacy is my very essence, then it's going to be nearly impossible to resolve the problem. There is no "space" available in which to resolve it! It is all taken up with the misidentification, "I-want-intimacy-but-I'm-afraid-to-get-that-close"—as if that is all I am. Further cluttering my internal space are a wealth of past experiences (content) that, in my view, reinforce my condition of fear of intimacy. Taken together, I've got a hermetically sealed problem with little room to move.

If I learn to move outside this misidentification so that I can view it, observe it, describe it, perhaps even write about it or paint it—in short, if I am the knower of the problem—then I am bigger than it. Simply put, it is not me. I am creating a larger context of selfhood that allows me to observe and disidentify at the same time. The problem no longer takes up all my inner space; it is surrounded by a context of perception and awareness that begins to diminish the valence of the problem.

There are many books about Eastern philosophy that discuss this vital principle of developing *context*. My forthcoming book, *Quantum Consciousness: The Discovery and Birth of Quantum Psychology: The Physics of Consciousness*, is a resource volume of approximately 100 different ways of disidentifying in order to experience oneself as context. Real transformation occurs when we move from being the content, or story, of our lives to being the context—or the space in which the life occurs.

You are not that which passes through your consciousness; you are not your thoughts, your emotions, your ideas, memories, fears. Deep Trance Phenomena are the means by which you shrink your *self* down to these limited states, by which you misidentify with the belief that "I'm a loser" or "I'm not smart enough" or "I can't get close." Once you shrink your sense of self down to become this belief or that belief by identifying with it, you find yourself completely isolated *inside* the experience. There is no context to provide perspective or resources. Anything that you identify with is going to limit you by blocking out any other experience.

Imagine your problem as a circle. The moment you identify yourself with the problem, in effect, you are stepping inside the circle. Once enclosed by the circle (the problematic state), all resources are impeded; they cannot pass through the boundary of the circle, which is comprised of the belief, "I am my problem." The moment you disidentify with the circle, its boundary becomes permeable and other options and resources begin to flow.

If there were only one key point to this entire book it would be that *you are not your problem; you are not your trance states which create your symptom. You are the creator and the knower or perceiver of your problem*. You are the being who chose particular responses to handle particular types of experiences; and you are the being who put those responses on automatic. That is the larger context that therapy must awaken in any person seeking a solution to a problem or a resolution of a symptom.

For Erickson, the concept of the unconscious mind played the pivotal role in therapeutic trance: it was the storehouse of resources and past experiences that could be drawn upon to bring about healing and resolution without the person's conscious awareness. In my approach, I find the concept of *context* much more useful because it does not compartmentalize the mind, as Erickson's conscious/unconscious split does. Furthermore, the concept of context empowers the individual by viewing the mind as an organic unity that continuously creates states of being. Erickson's conscious/unconscious split, on the other hand, tends to idealize one part (the unconscious) as the savior while making the other part (the conscious mind) the enemy or at least the annoying interloper.

There are parts of yourself you choose to be conscious of, and there are parts you choose not to "see"—all depending upon the twists and turns of your past experiences in combination with your own sensory-perceptual preferences and temperament. Potentially, you could choose to view any aspect of your past experience. This is what being aware of context gives you: It empowers you with the awareness of the scope of your own mind.

I always think of this in terms of an image. The mind is a library, and what you choose to experience in the course of a day is a product of you, the being behind the transient states of consciousness, standing in the library and retrieving particular sections. If you so chose, you can take the flashlight of your awareness into the history section, or the relationship section, or the business section, or the body section, and retrieve whatever you need. The point is, all the material is always there, but it can *only be viewed if you choose to focus your mental flashlight on it.*

When I talk about shrinking your focus of attention (or misidentifying) so that the "you behind the trance" goes unnoticed, versus the concept of perceiving the full context of who you really are, I find that people often need some kind of image to make it more tangible. For me, the image is one of an infinite night sky, alit with thousands of planets and thousands of stars (the context). Into this vast dimension steps the limiting identification that "I am the planet called depression" (or whatever). By shrinking your focus of attention down to just one particle in this immense expanse, *and assuming that's all you are*, you create the very problem or symptom by which you feel overpowered. In fact, *you* are the knower, and your Deep Trance Phenomena are the vehicle of your consuming identification with the planet called depression.

So, to reiterate, the beginning stage of therapy involves pointing out the misidentification and helping the person observe her own process. This in itself gives the person an introductory taste of separating from the problem, for the perceiver is separate from that which is perceived. The moment an individual steps into the observer mode, she is expanding her own context and beginning to dismantle her misidentifications.

In order for a therapist to be able to help a client discover himself as the knower, the therapist (needless to say) needs to be beyond his own Deep Trance Phenomena. In other words, he needs to be well versed in the practice of self-observation, well able to "catch" his own misidentifications, and familiar with the sensation of shifting among identities rather than identifying with them.

Perhaps an example from my own life will demonstrate this point.

About a year and a half ago I was in a very intense relationship with a woman. I thought things were going along wonderfully when, one night, I received a phone call from her. She said that "it was over"!

With those three words I felt myself deluged with anger and hurt. For half an hour I ranted and raved, feeling desolated and abandoned. Then, a shift occurred and I "remembered" all I knew about how such unpleasant states are created. I got a very clear picture of having gone to my mental library and turned my flashlight of awareness onto the section called "Rejection," whereupon I retrieved all the standard responses I had learned for that experience—and fully identified with them. By identifying with them, I was re-creating them in present time. Worse, the problem was automatically enlarged and amplified: by going into the library of my mind and retrieving *all past experiences* labeled "Rejection," I was experiencing a lifetime of accumulated events rather than simply the one in the present moment. Past was melded to present, with the future thrown in for dramatic effect ("This is the story of my life" theme).

I then felt a tangible sensation of expansion occur as the misidentifications fell away. I let the body responses run their own course, realizing that particular sensations don't have to mean "rejection" or "humiliation" or "hurt." *I* am the one who gives sensations one label or another. So I observed as my body experienced flushing, rapid breathing, and heart palpitations. I noticed how the waves of emotion I had been calling "rejection" also frequently accompanied sexual arousal, or excitement at a Celtics game, or any number of other pleasant experiences. I realized that we not only choose our responses, but perhaps more importantly, we choose the labels we give them. A rose by any other name *is not* a rose.

Witnessing

The moment you step outside of your problem to observe it, you create a larger context for it. Observing or *witnessing* thus becomes a key activity of therapy. I first came across the concept of witnessing in Eastern literature—in the *Bhagavad Gita*—where Krishna is described as the "Eternal Witness" (Jnaneshvari, 1962) Krishna gives counsel to poor Arjuna, who represents all of us normal humans in life crises. Krishna teaches Arjuna how to interact with his states of consciousness so that they do not rule him by developing an awareness of his true nature as witness. The entire *Bhagavad Gita* revolves around the concept of the Eternal Witness as the means of disentangling ourselves from worldly perils. Indeed, in Chapter 13 entitled "The Field and the Knower of the Field: The Yoga of Distinction," Krishna defines the field as the body and repeatedly emphasizes the need to know the knower of the field, because the body-field is where experiences are experienced.

From my Eastern perspective, it seemed to me that therapeutic trance was really a Western way of trying to establish a witnessing consciousness. In the hypnosis literature, the term *dissociation* is used to describe trance processes whereby one part of the individual steps back and looks at the overall situation. When dissociation is used therapeutically in hypnotic work, it is most often described as a means of splitting off or "depotentiating" the conscious mind from the unconscious (Erickson, Rossi, & Rossi, 1976; Erickson & Rossi, 1979). As mentioned previously, the conscious mind is viewed as the interloper; the unconscious mind as the bearer of all the fruits.

On one hand, I view dissociation as an automatic defense

whereby, for example, you experience yourself floating at the top of the room in order to defend yourself against a molest. On the other hand, dissociation means *not associating with*. When you can choose to fuse or associate with and choose to *not* associate with (disassociation), you have developed the ability to choose or not to choose to witness the content of your experience.

Witnessing, furthermore, is characterized by a subtle but important shift in focus. It does not involve a sense of splitting or depotentiating different regions of the mind. It is a unified experience of perception that allows and embraces without limiting and shrinking one's focus of attention. Emphasis is placed on the awareness of the self or being behind the ongoing activity, rather than on portioning out and labeling different aspects of mental functioning.

Expanded Contexts of Healing

Witnessing can be used to bring about what we might think of as four stages whereby context is increasingly expanded in a manner that naturally results in therapeutic resolutions of problems or symptoms.

STEP 1: Expanding the Context to Include the Body. Often, physical symptoms are experienced by the sufferer as having a strange autonomy in the body. A stomach ache, for example, narrows one's focus down to the problematic stomach, as if it were a dissociated but truant offender; the rest of the body is experienced as separate from the uncomfortable area.

In Gestalt therapy a problem is created when the "figure" is separated from the "ground." In the following example, the figure (stomach ache) is separated from the ground (body). By using suggestion to reconnect the figure to the ground (expand the context of the person's experience) via sensation, a new experience begins to develop.

"As you continue to notice the sensations in your stomach—and I don't know exactly how you experience those particular sensations—you might experience them as vibrations. . . .You might experience them as subtle movements. . . .You've got a right hand; you've got a left hand. Now I don't know which hand you might experience sensations in first, whether it is that one over there or the one over here, but as you notice which one it is, you might notice that sensations are occurring there, and I don't know how sensations move. . . .But I do know that sensations can, will, and do move from your right hand or from your left hand. . . .up into your elbow. Or maybe just to your wrist. Or perhaps just to the middle of your forearm. . . .And I don't know how you will feel a subtle warmth, a sensation, a tingling, or exactly how you experience these different sensibilities. . . .But you can experience them.

"And as you experience it even more, it can move up the center of your arm, over the top of your shoulder, into your neck. . . .You have sensations and pulsations and vibrations and accumulations of energy throughout your body that you can. . .continue to enjoy."

If the presenting problem is, for example, "a feeling of sadness over the death of my father," I would work in the same way to expand the *context* of the bodily sensations. I would ask the client to tell me where in her body she felt the sadness. She might say, "I feel sad all over." I would ask, "In your earlobes? In your ankles? In your shoulder blades?" "No," she would answer, "I guess it's mainly in my chest."

The purpose of this expansion technique is not to deny what the person is currently experiencing but to ignite latent resources to facilitate the healthy processing of that experience.

Axiom: Reconnecting the experience of the symptom to the entire "field" of the body automatically expands the awareness, thus shifting the subjective experience of the symptom.

STEP 2: Expanding the Context to Include the Self. Connecting both the symptom and the body back to a sense of "I" or ego self is the next step. In most cases, the symptom originally was dissociated from the body as a means of protecting the individual from experiencing something he or she was not willing to experience. Establishing a reconnection between symptom, body and self creates the context for an experience to be felt and processed, which in turn ensures future integration and ego development. It is through the expansion and reconnection of the "I" back to the body which shifts the body back into alignment with the self.

Let's continue with the stomach ache example. To reestablish a sense of "I-ness" or selfhood, I would begin by asking the person to breathe and look at me. I establish intense eye contact as a rapid means of constellating their *I*-contact. Typically, this I-contact is paradoxically preceded by an experience of dissociation of "spacing out," which is immediately utilized in the giving of suggestions:

"And as you begin to space out and notice the stomach ache, you can. . .continue to breathe and look at me."

Utilizing the dissociation while placing it in a wholly new context—"breathe and look at me"—usually triggers all the Deep Trance Phenomena in the person's lifetime repertoire of defenses. I call these "pop-up trances," because that is exactly what they seem to do!

The client continues to space out even more, to the point of blocking me out of her vision.

"And as everything continues to fog, just breathe and look at me."

Allowing her to dissociate—even utilizing and facilitating it—allows me to view her entire symptom complex. In essence, her Deep Trance Phenomena march out to protect her "I" from directly relating to me as she "breathes and looks at me." I observe these trance states and assemble the ingredients, like you would a cake. First comes the stomach ache, then comes the spaciness and dissociation, then comes fogged vision, then comes numbness in limbs.

Now I can begin to reassociate the person's sense of self, which has been dispersed via Deep Trance Phenomena, with suggestions that might go as follow:

"Now I don't know what image might be valuable for you to. . .experience directly, but I do know that it will be interesting as well as surprising to notice. . .notice. . .notice what image might. . .remind you of the you. . .you need."

At this point an image emerges—a mountain, a tiger, a dove, a bear—that is representative of the lost "I." I then ask the client to place this image in the part of the body it seems to "belong." This placement connects the "I" to the body.

Continually asking the client to "breathe and look at me" is a physical means of expanding her awareness. Furthermore, it allows her to move from an intrapersonal trance to an interpersonal trance with me. Trance work is done with eyes open, which I have found is essential if the trance work is to become integrated in life: Life is not lived with eyes closed and a floating sensation of spaciness; it is lived *in direct contact* with our surrounding environment.

Requiring the contact of breathing and looking at me demands an intimacy which eventually—after all the defensive trance phenomena have popped up to protect it—constellates the person's "I-hood." Now, everybody is co-existing: all the Deep Trance Phenomena *as well as* the "I." When the person entered the session, her trance phenomena were on automatic and the "I" was thoroughly dissociated or "spaced out."

Let's take another example. A woman I worked with, who had been sexually abused as a child, was plagued by chronic back pain. Whenever she was in a sexual situation, her back and pelvic area would respond with sensations of pain. Consequently, she did not have sex.

In looking at how she created this traumatized response in present time, I saw that it began by her focusing all her attention to that area—she was aware solely of the sensations in her back and pelvis. Secondly, she dissociated from the experience; her self or "I" would go into trances of dissociation and amnesia—which were the same trance phenomena she had developed as a child to handle the experience of being made to have sex with her stepfather.

In reversing this response pattern, I began by expanding her context of the sensation of her symptoms by using hypnotic suggestions that put her in touch with all the other regions of her body that were not in pain. Her body could then be experienced as an organic whole—a physical organism with unity and integrity. Next, I worked with her to bring this expanded body context into relationship with her sense of self:

"And as you continue to feel the sensations in your pelvis and lower back, I wonder how long it would take for the sensations to move. . .move. . .move into your chest, arms, neck, and head. . .not to mention your legs and feet."

These suggestions connect the pelvic and lower back sensations to the whole body so that the figure (the pelvis) is no longer disconnected from the ground (the body).

Next I asked for an image that would reconnect her sense of self, her "I-ness," to her body:

"And as you continue to breathe and look at me, it might be interesting to notice an image or symbol that represents an expanded or deeper self. I don't know if it will be a river or a mountain, a dog or a lion, but you might. . .let me know when it emerges."

Once the image is retrieved, you again ask the client to place it in the appropriate part of the body, thus completing the integration of self with body.

Axiom: Reconnecting the symptom and body with a sense of self or "I" shifts the body back into alignment with the self. The addition of the self further expands the context of the experience and prepares the individual for the activity of witnessing.

STEP 3: Expanding the Context to Include the Social Network. Now that the symptom has been reintegrated with the body, which has a strong sense of "I-ness," the newly expanded "I" needs to be integrated into the larger social setting from which it has been split off. To state this more pragmatically, the client and I have shared this joint trance experience—but how can she relate that experience to her outer world? How can she integrate the intense two-person exchange of the therapy room with her daily life?

I begin the process of expanding the client's awareness to encompass the social network by evoking resources within the person: An image, metaphor, or symbol representing the "I" is experienced by the individual in the mind's eye, and then generalized to include or embrace a social context that is reflective of his or her actual life situation. I might say, for example:

"I don't know exactly when or how, but at some point your unconscious mind is going to give you an image, an unconscious image, an image of integration, a symbol of your deep Self. It might be a mountain. . .or a river. . .or an animal. . .or perhaps just a shape—and this symbol will help you to percolate, circulate, accumulate, and integrate all these particular ideas into your daily life."

This particular client saw Mount Vesuvius in her mind's eye. Next I asked her, "Where would you like to put that image in your physical body?"

She answered after a few moments, "In my heart."

"And as you continue to breathe and look at me, you are seeing and feeling and hearing Mount Vesuvius right inside your heart."

Now that a resource has been evoked and vividly experienced physically, in the body, I want to expand its connection outside of the client to embrace, eventually, her problem area. First I suggest to her that she also see her image simultaneously inside me as well as inside herself. This is then extended to include any number of people, culminating with whomever the problem centers around:

> "And, you know, the checker at your market can also have a Mount Vesuvius in his heart. . .and your dry cleaner. . .and your hairdresser. Why shouldn't they? And the symbol of Mount Vesuvius can also be held in Harold's heart. . .and as you look at Harold the next time you feel that old tension beginning to build, you can feel your own Mount Vesuvius in your heart, and you can see Harold's Mount Vesuvius in his heart. . .Your image, your beautiful, deep, connecting symbol can be equally inside other people in your life, so that you can be a part of the relationship with them, and at the same time, apart from it."

This concept of being a part of and a part from a relationship simultaneously has been developed and taught by Gilligan (1987). In Jungian terms, I am offering the client a specific way of projecting positive qualities (qualities that feel good to her) that will help interrupt her pattern of negative projections (experiencing the other person as bearing unpleasant, harmful, or critical qualities). In Zen terms, I am opening the door to a personal experience of unity, of oneness, that inevitably broadens a person's context and evokes a wealth of coping resources.

Axiom: Connecting the self back to the present life context further shifts the symptom structure while continuing to expand the person's inner awareness.

STEP 4: Expanding the Context to Include the Inner Witness. The least addressed and yet most important aspect of therapeutic work, I believe, is the cultivation of the person's "inner knower": that part within which holds or contains all experiences—what I have called the witness. Say, for example, that you are embroiled in an internal conflict of polarized desires: "I want a career," "I don't want a career." The development of witnessing expands the internal context in a way that allows both sides of the conflict (I want/I don't want) to exist simultaneously. Also, it points to the *you*, the knower of the conflict.

Let me say at this point that all four of these steps overlap. There is no set hierarchy; no rigid lines of demarcation. Witnessing is involved in all of the steps, but is particularly emphasized in Step 4 as a means of consolidating the overall exercise and hopefully interweaving the activity of witnessing into a person's ongoing consciousness. An example of what can be said to evoke this experience might be:

> "I wonder what it's like to witness your physical body right now, the movements of your jaw as you swallow, your eyes moving in changing directions, the small movements of your thighs on the chair as you shift your position, the position of your hands in your lap, perhaps a moment of laughter. And as you begin to notice it, to just look at it from a subtle distance, it is nice to know that you can expand a little bit past it. And as you experience that witnessing state, you will notice. . . ."

These kinds of suggestions help put the person in touch with the sensation of witnessing. Another way of concretizing the witnessing experience is by suggesting an image of that inner witnessing space, just as we evoked a symbol of "I" in relation to a social network. Now another symbolic resource can come to consciousness as a means of visualizing and personalizing the "witness within."

> "And as you notice that part of you that is witnessing or watching, there might be some kind of a symbol, or an idea, or a picture pop up that emphasizes, figurizes, illuminizes, visualizes that inner witness."

One woman I worked with got a clear image of a rainbow as a symbol of her inner space of witnessing. I continued:

> "And I don't know exactly how many rainbows you can see over. . .around. . .through. I don't know where you'll even see that. But it will be interesting to see how often you do experience those particular rainbows over you, around you,

or through you. . . and over, around, through me. . .and other people whom you encounter. And it's nice to know that you can. . .will. . .do experience them equally."

The first symbol the client was asked to create was one of the deep self—the "I" that organizes one's psychological being. This additional symbol is of the witness that can observe even that "I."

Setting Intentions

Another primary task of the therapist in the beginning session is to discern his own as well as the client's *intentions* and *counter-intentions*. This is done by inquiring within oneself and asking the client to do the same. Too often, problems and obstacles arise between therapist and client because they are not aligned at the level of intention. Clients end up feeling frustrated and misunderstood, while therapists generally label the client as "resistant."

For example, a woman comes to me and describes a chronically dysfunctional relationship with her husband. She concludes with the statement of her intention, which is "But I really want to stay with my husband. I want to find a way to work things out." Meanwhile, a part of my psyche has the opposite response, which translates as a counter-intention of "I think you should leave the bastard."

Instead of trying to get the client to see it my way, or pushing down my internal response and forcing myself to see it my client's way, *I will acknowledge and utilize this counter-intention*, just as I acknowledge and utilize whatever the client presents. Without necessarily verbalizing my counter-intention, I would simply notice it, allow it to be there, and expand to include it.

Sometimes a counter-intention within the client will need to be brought out into the open before therapy can really proceed. I worked with a 27-year-old man who had been heavily into drugs since he was 14. He had seen a dozen different therapists by the time he was referred to me. His opening statement was, "I want to quit using drugs." I simply didn't believe him and told him so. He began to give me reasons why he wanted to quit using drugs, and I would tell him why he didn't need to. Finally, 45 minutes later, he said, "You know, part of me really doesn't want to quit drugs." Acknowledging both his intention and his counter-intention cleared the space for the therapy. Rather then pretend to do some kind of drug intervention therapy espousing the virtues of abstinence—to which he would have responded, "Fuck you man, I'm not going to quit"—I focused on simply allowing both sides of the drug experience to co-exist.

Horner (1988) has described intention as being "the highest power a being has; everything springs from intention." In the Buddhist point of view, *intention* is recognized as preceding movement or thought, and is likened to an impulse. In Vipassana meditation, one can begin to observe or witness intentions prior to body movements or verbal interactions.

Erickson, in his inimitably mischievous way, tells a story of that humorously expresses his view of intention (Rossi & Ryan, 1991). He was standing in a formal queue (with Margaret Mead) to thank a hostess for the lovely dinner he had enjoyed. He watched as the guests preceding him said all the right things in all the right ways, and then he decided to conduct his own "field experiment" on the spot: When his turn came, he ever so courteously, so grandly, thanked the hostess for the lovely dinner of *horses' tail*, and could he have the recipe? Oh, certainly, she replied, she would be most happy to give him that recipe! For Erickson, the actual words he spoke were never as important as the meaning and intent he ascribed to them.

The role of intention in therapy is preeminent. Only when intentions as well as counter-intentions are acknowledged can the therapist and client become mutually aligned in a cooperative therapeutic venture. Setting the intention creates the context for change—and no change can occur without a space first being cleared for it.

If I, as the therapist, acknowledge any counter-intentions I am experiencing in relation to the client, I am going to have a free flow of my associations and responses. If I block those parts of myself, I'm not going to have a free flow, *and* I will be teaching the client that those blocked parts are unacceptable.

Let's say I begin to feel angry in a session. If I resist that anger I will also give an unconscious message to my client that says: *It's not okay to be angry*. If I resist my feeling of stuckness about what to do next, then I'm telling my client, in effect, that he should resist his own feeling of stuckness of his life. That is why I feel safe acknowledging any thought, feeling, association, emotion, or counter-intention that pops up in me; to do otherwise would only pollute the therapeutic environment.

Just as the client needs to be introduced to the concept of expanding his or her own inner context, so does the therapist. I need to learn how to allow all of my perceptions and responses *without identifying myself as them.*

Moving Beyond an Identity as "Therapist"

Being a therapist is as much (if not more) about my own growth as it is about my clients'. We are present as equals. Unfortunately, a sense of equality is not generally taught in supervision. Rather, we are encouraged and even pressured into rigid role definitions that are supposed to protect us while somehow helping our clients.

Pioneer family therapist Carl Whitaker (1989; Whitaker & Malone, 1987) first attempted to dispel this polarity by introducing the concept of "co-transference" (as opposed to the traditional dyad, transference/countertransference). His message was, We're all in this together, we all project on each other, we all try to hide, we all try to manipulate, we are all trying to grow. Now in his mid-seventies, Whitaker uses his lecturing circuit to "go crazy as the patient" for the audience. Whitaker's best times occur when he fully allows himself to "share his own craziness."

Perhaps the most profound way for a person earning a living as a therapist to expand his or her inner context is to integrate and own the understanding that *there is no difference between the therapist and the client.* In a training group in which I was discussing this idea I was asked, "Then, how do you know who's the therapist and who's the client?"

My answer: "The person who gets paid is the therapist."

That drew laughs, but I really did not intend it to be a humorous communication. On the contrary, I was quite serious. The invisible but potent barrier separating therapist from client is one of the largest obstacles to personal growth any therapist will encounter.

We all know that therapy is more than technique; we all know, at least in our heads, that *our being, our essence*, is far more important than the execution of any technique, Ericksonian or otherwise. Being fully present for the person labeled "client" is the most therapeutic thing I can offer. But what does that mean, in psychological terms?

As mentioned, because of the training we receive, most of us as therapists tend to create an identity called "therapist." Our selfhood then gets funneled into that identity, which serves as a limitation as well as a sanctuary—we can hide behind this role any time we choose. And we can't possibly grow if we are hiding behind a role and behaving in ways that correspond to our mental images of what a therapist/psychologist looks like, dresses like, talks like, and so forth. Worse, we tend to put our therapist identity on automatic, which means it runs fairly rampant in our lives. And, as will be elaborated later, each identity has a counter-identity underneath it, so we generally feel compelled to put everyone we relate to in a counter-role as client. Stated more bluntly, if we create identities called "therapist," then we have to have clients! Friends, relatives, spouses, and post office clerks are all viewed and responded to from the narrow vantage point of our identity as "therapist." Furthermore, we tend to try to fit every client into a "model"—whichever one we have adopted—without acknowledging who he or she is beyond the role or symptom being presented. In a nutshell, a therapist's identity is a trance state because it narrows and shrinks the focus of attention. The therapist's identity might be a beneficial one, but nonetheless, if a therapist identifies and limits himself to this identity, he is greatly limiting his resources and inhibiting his own growth process.

The much cherished goal of "rapport" can often be no more than the collusion between therapist and client to agree upon their identities and produce the behavior that manifests that. If you come to see me for therapy and I create the identity of "brilliant interpreter," then it is likely that you will create a counter-identity as "dumb, helpless client" who tells me how much I know and who is very responsive to everything I say. That is called rapport.

More importantly, therapists who take on helper identities are often denying their own feelings of helplessness. The helper identify then projects the helpless identity onto the client. If the client doesn't "buy into" this role, he or she is usually labeled resistant. Therapists often attempt to fit the client into their model without acknowledging who they are beyond the roles and the symptoms.

If, however, you as the client don't play by these unspoken identity rules and disagree with me, or tell me you see things very differently, or even openly challenge me, then you will probably be labeled "resistant" or worse. Similarly, if I as the therapist refuse to accommodate the identity you expect me to manifest, you may label me "incompetent" or worse.

It has taken me a long time to learn to *be*—and that includes allowing the experience of not-knowing. When I feel stuck in a session and don't know how to proceed or even what to say, I say so. I focus on the sensations of not knowing and continue to breathe with it. In Erickson's terms, I utilize it—but it has now become a lifestyle rather than just a technique. Erickson's utilization principles coincide beautifully with Eastern concepts of meditation: do not discard, dissociate from, or resist anything. Observe. . .allow. . . embrace.

Learning to Spot Your Own Deep Trance Phenomena

Unless you can observe and identify your own deep trances, there is no way you will be able to spot them in clients. In searching for a way to learn how to do this with myself, I made use of a meditation-like environment with which I was already quite familiar as a way of focusing my attention on my own Deep Trance Phenomena. I would sit quietly for a period of time each day, observe the thoughts and feelings that arose and subsided, and begin to label them in terms of trance states.

For instance, watching my thoughts move into concerns about future events meant I was experiencing pseudo-orientation in time; the emergence of angry feelings from the past usually meant I was age-regressing; and the sensation of feeling there was not enough time for me indicated time distortion. I would notice when my physical environment began to fade visually and register that as negative hallucination; I would notice which parts of my body were present via sensation and which were disconnected and dissociated. And so on.

I carefully structured my initial learnings by proceeding in a slow and methodical fashion made possible by the meditation-like environment I created for myself. Once I felt some facility under these controlled circumstances, I moved my awareness out into the more chaotic world. I began catching myself in various trance states throughout the day, both alone and while interacting, and simply tracked them. I spotted my trances, as it were, and noticed definite patterns and preferences. My favorite Deep Trance Phenomenon, which I could fall into almost any time, was negative hallucination: whenever a situation or person would begin to irritate me, I would simply stop seeing. Your preference might be dissociation, confusion, or age-regression—it all depends on your personal past history and what worked best in your family.

At first, as with any learning process, there is a certain sense of awkward effort and concentration required to begin perceiving and identifying Deep Trance Phenomena in yourself and your clients. I remember watching a client and thinking laboriously: "He looks like he's starting to space out—ah-ha—he's dissociating. . .now there is a light film over his eyes—oh, that must be negative hallucination. . .he's worrying about a business meeting two weeks away—that's pseudo-orientation in time." Within five minutes of intense observation, I was exhausted.

It is certainly possible to get compulsive in the learning process and end up feeling as if you are tramping around in a marshland of confusion. If you feel that confusion coming over you, sit back, *breathe deeply*, and *just notice what the client is giving you*. You don't have to think; you don't have to figure it out. *Just notice what the client is giving you.*

The primary purpose of this book revolves around learning how to identify and work with Deep Trance Phenomena: first, as a therapist, to be able to work with your clients by noticing and altering their trances; secondly and more importantly is to be able to spot and alter your own trances. Ironically, accomplishing the first purpose is contingent upon first accomplishing the second.

In my psychotherapy training programs, therapists regularly lament: "I can't see the subject's age regression, I feel powerless"; "I can't see the negative hallucination"; or, "I can't understand how to do this. . .I'm confused." Each time my answer is essentially the same: *You cannot spot someone else's trances until you can spot your own.* Without the foundation of self-knowledge in this area, you will find yourself feeling helpless (age regression) as you fail to spot your client's negative hallucination because you yourself are negatively hallucinating. Or you will not understand what your client is saying because you are caught in your own Deep Trance Phenomenon of confusion.

Based on my personal experience in learning how to spot my own Deep Trance Phenomena, I developed three progressive exercises that can be done sequentially. Notice that Exercises 2 and 3 repeat the steps of the preceeding exercise. In a forthcoming book, *Quantum Consciousness*, approximately one hundred techniques are presented to deepen this gradient of understanding.

Exercise No. 1

Step 1: Sit or lie down in a comfortable position.

Step 2: Begin to watch your mind closely, noticing how it keeps throwing up ideas, thoughts, pictures, and internal dialogues.

Step 3: Detach yourself and simply observe the comings and goings of the ideas, thoughts, pictures, and internal dialogues.

Exercise No. 2

Step 1: Sit or lie down in a comfortable position.

Step 2: Begin to watch your mind closely, noticing how it keeps throwing up (no pun intended) ideas, thoughts, pictures, and internal dialogues.

Step 3: Detach yourself and simply observe the comings and goings of the ideas, thoughts, pictures, and internal dialogues.

Step 4: Begin to label each thought or picture or idea as a Deep Trance Phenomenon. For example, if your mind is going back to the past, label it *age regression*. If your mind is going into the future, label it *pseudo-orientation in time*. When you feel spacey, label it *dissociation*. If you get dreamy, label it *hypnotic dreaming*. And so forth. In this way you begin to differentiate specific Deep Trance Phenomena out of the diffusive mass of trance states.

Exercise No. 3

Step 1: Sit or lie down in a comfortable position.

Step 2: Begin to watch your mind closely, noticing how it keeps throwing up ideas, thoughts, pictures, and internal dialogues.

Step 3: Detach yourself and simply observe the comings and goings of the ideas, thoughts, pictures, and internal dialogues.

Step 4: Begin to label each thought or picture or idea as a Deep Trance Phenomenon. For example, if your mind is going back to the past, label it *age regression*. If your mind is going into the future, label it *pseudo-orientation in time*. When you feel spacey, label it *dissociation*. If you get dreamy, label it *hypnotic dreaming*. And so forth. In this way you begin to differentiate specific Deep Trance Phenomena out of the diffusive mass of trance states.

Step 5: Knowingly, consciously, intentionally create or produce the Deep Trance Phenomenon that is already occurring. For example, let's say you hear an internal voice that says, "Life is hard." Label it *posthypnotic suggestion*. Now intentionally create the voice saying, "Life is hard" several times. Then let it go. If a picture from the past "pops up" (age regression), internally create several copies of the picture, look at them, and then let them go. If you feel your body going numb (*sensory distortion*), knowingly create the numbness several times. If you notice your mind is beginning to fantasize (*hypnotic dreaming*), consciously re-create that experience several times.

Ultimately, these exercises will produce several effects:

(1) You will be able to spot your own trances.
(2) You will notice other people's trances.
(3) You will begin to identify yourself as the observer or witness of the comings and goings of different deep trance states.
(4) You will begin to experience that you are the creator of these trance phenomena and, consequently, beyond their effects.

The ultimate outcome of these three exercises is an encompassing understanding that you are not your trance phenomena; that you created your trances initially as a defense and then, in essence, put them on automatic; and, finally, that by intentionally creating Deep Trance Phenomena in present time, you gain control over them and they disappear, leaving you with your *self*. What you are left with is *you:* the observer and creator of your experience.

7

Age Regression

Whether we care to admit it or not, most of us experience spurts of age regression on a fairly frequent basis. If only for 30 seconds after being reprimanded by a boss, spouse, or friend, we all know how it feels to cascade back in time psychologically and emotionally. The young wife who curls up on her husband's lap to entice him into buying her a new dress is the same little girl who first learned to crawl onto Daddy's lap and "be cute" in order to get what she wanted. Age regression grants the little girl of yesteryear the automatic response of using what worked for her in the past in present time.

The problem is that the adult in present time *automatically* and *unknowingly* age regresses to get what she wants. Often, she feels powerless and resents the lack of respect she receives from her partner. She might feel misunderstood, unseen, and even alienated. All these psychoemotional states are glued together by an unknowing adult utilizing age regression.

Age regression is probably the most widely experienced Deep Trance Phenomenon and almost always a contributor in the presenting problem or symptom. Erickson (1980) defined age regression as "the tendency on the part of the personality to revert to some method or form of expression belonging to an earlier phase of personality development" (p. 104). I see it more as the interpolation of a past, time-frozen experience over present reality whereby the individual cannot adequately experience present time. Actually, Erickson gets quite close to this view in describing how "mental states can be induced that are unrelated to immediate reality but are, so far as can be determined, actual reactivation of mental states previously experienced and uninfluenced by mental patterns acquired subsequent to the original experiences" (p. 105).

Erickson tended to focus on dramatic examples of age regression underlying usually severe episodes of psychological dysfunction. I have become amazed at how pervasive age regression is in symptomatology in general. It seems to be the most common "ingredient" in the symptom "cake"—that is, the most frequent Deep Trance Phenomenon in the cluster of phenomena comprising problems and symptoms. Indeed, you can even presuppose the presence of regression in any symptom, for such a symptom must have a *time frozen* quality to it that permits its repetition.

Being stuck in a past "place" creates the guidelines for current interpersonal limitations. Age regression creates developmental gaps that interrupt, impede, and/or undermine adult functioning.

As with all Deep Trance Phenomena, age regression was originally created as a result of interpersonal interactions which, for whatever reasons, the child was not able to integrate. In order *not* to integrate an experience—in essence, to *resist* it—the child freezes his body by tightening his muscles and holding his breath. This physiological pattern may then become the somatic basis for an automatic response—an *intra*personal self-to-self trance that endures for decades to come.

For example, Dad has a terrible habit of telling Mikie that he'll never make it—that he'll be as much a failure as his father is. Statements to that effect become part of Mikie's daily psychological menu, and he learns to deflect them by freezing his body and holding his breath.

The formation of *hypnotic identities* and *oppositional identities* is discussed in detail in Chapters 10 and 19. For now, it is enough to say that Mikie begins to fuse with the experience called "I'm-a-failure-just-like-Dad," and this fusion is held together in a trance identity that defines how he views himself. He also begins to form a counter-identity of "I-can-do-anything-I-set-my-mind-on-doing." Out of the counter-identity, Mikie is driven to achieve. By age eight he is already being called a "super-achiever"; by age 15, he's getting straight A's and holding down two part-time jobs; by age 21 he's passing his bar exams; by age 25 he's a junior partner in a prestigious law firm. And so on.

The fascinating part of this story is the invisible web of deep trance dynamics that make it possible. There are two parts to this web. In the first part, much of the "steam" for Michael-the-Adult's successful law career is coming from the "solution" Little Mikie created in response to his own discomfort and psychological pain. Since that solution (a trance identity called "I-can-do-anything-I-set-my-mind-on-doing") was created during childhood, it requires an ongoing age-regressed state to maintain it. What that means is, Little Mikie is always present within Michael-the-Adult as a needy little child running around trying to prove himself worthy.

In part two of the web, Michael-the-Adult unwittingly holds in his consciousness the painful trance identity called "I'm-a-failure-just-like-Dad" he originally created as a child. He literally fuses with or "becomes" Dad again and again. *He has to keep his mental picture of failure present in his mind in order to promise himself that he'll never be like that!* The ultimate double bind is that his continued achievement as Michael-the-Adult is contingent upon the promptings of Little Mikie's "I'm-a-failure" identity.

In issues of sexual abuse, more often than not the child fuses with the perpetrator. At some level the child becomes and holds the perpetrator in his consciousness while simultaneously holding the victim consciousness. This explains the psychodynamics of why victims of sexual abuse become perpetrators in later life.

Let's take a closer look at how something that is born out of an *interpersonal* dynamic can function for long periods of time as an *intrapersonal* force.

Think back to the last time you lost your temper with someone. Bring the picture up the forefront of your awareness, and imagine a slow-motion special effect as you watch the incident unfold in your mind's eye. At first, you are dealing interpersonally with the other person; there is a sense of your*self*, and a clear sense of *other*. As the anger escalates, however, the trance lines blur considerably, and if you watch really closely, you can see the interpersonal trance dissipate into a purely *intra*psychic one. It is no longer you and the other person in a self-to-other anger trance; it has become a self-to-self trance in which you are recreating an experience from your childhood. Your focus shrinks even further as you glide out of present time (a 1991 trance) into the past (a 1955 trance). The particular type of *intrapersonal* trance you move into will depend on the altered state of consciousness you created as a child to defend yourself.

Another way to understand this is that as a four-year-old child, say, a violation occurs triggering anger; at age seven, another violation with more repressed anger; at age 12, the same. When at age 40 the adult is violated, the anger experienced is way out of proportion to the current trigger. Why? Because the event at age 40 catalyzes all earlier violations. This is age-regressed anger whereby the adult "retrieves" the age-regressed child and re-experiences it in present time—instantaneously, out of time.

Understanding that both *intra-* and *inter*personal dynamics co-exist in any individual bridges a longstanding dispute in the field of psychotherapy in which one school seeks to prove that all interactions are context-dependent (the family therapists), while another passionately asserts that the individual is the only source of lasting change (depth psychotherapists). Another way of integrating the intrapersonal with the interpersonal is to understand that individuals create trances in response to *inter*personal contexts, which they then internalize as a self-to-self trance. In other words, they are having an interpersonal interaction in an intrapersonal context.

I have found that pathology as well as health is a product of the combination of both intrapsychic processes and interpersonal dynamics. Family therapists tend to lose sight of the fact that each person has an internal world which he or she recreates in present time. Depth psychotherapists tend to minimize the pivotal role played by all "significant others" in a child's life; they also minimize the reality that behavior can change by changing the present-time context or interactions. Here we are going to make use of both sides of the coin and begin to realize in the process how little difference there is between what we encapsulate as "inner" and what we assign to "outer."

Principles Underlying Treatment

Most Deep Trance Phenomena come in clusters; you usually won't see *just* an age regression or *just* a dissociation or *just* a time distortion. Rather, a latticework of altered states of consciousness is interwoven over time, which you as the therapist will begin to discern, differentiate, utilize, and interrupt. For now, we will continue to focus on one trance state as if it were the sole component of the symptomatology.

> *Axiom: Vary the Deep Trance Phenomenon underlying the symptom and the symptom will lose its strength.*

Discovering and identifying the Deep Trance Phenomenon that is creating the symptom is the first task of the therapist. The next step follows naturally: to witness and fully appreciate the client's selected Deep Trance Phenomenon as his or her gift to you. Let yourself "be with the client," become familiar with the client's unique version of the symptom, recognize it as a masterful creation. As the therapist you take the attitude toward the client of: "Teach me how you create your symptom. What exactly do you do to get the outcome called a *problem*?" In this way the client is actually the teacher and demonstrator; the therapist has to remain willing to learn from the client.

Now you can begin to alter the symptomatic trance in a number of ways. The client is constructing her current reality by altering present time via age regression. You help her to construct a different reality (one without the symptom or problem) by altering the age regression in present time. I have already discussed how my approach to altering the Deep Trance Phenomena underlying symptomatology differs from Erickson's technique of pattern interruption in which he used induced therapeutic trance states to interrupt or block the occurrence of the symptom. Since, in my view, clients bring their trance state with them—and *that* is the problem—there is no need to induce a competing trance state, even if it is more comfortable than their self-created one.

Evoking Reassociations. As mentioned previously, Deep Trance Phenomena are put on "automatic" and function in a stimulus-response mode: *Stimulus A* invariably triggers *Response "B."*

Furthermore, the range of territory, so to speak, covered by the stimulus-response pattern becomes larger and larger as the original Stimulus A is generalized to encompass (or contaminate) more and more. Thus, Father's angry reprimands, which were the original Stimulus A, gradually become generalized to include. . .all male authority figures. . .all men with black moustaches. . .all people who drink alcohol, and so on.

So, as a therapist you begin with a rigid stimulus-response pattern that usually has a wide circumference. For example, a client who was molested as a young child by her "Uncle Henry" had learned to fixate on his left eye as a way of distracting herself from what was really going on. Now, as an adult, the traumatic eye stimulus generalized to all men with whom she attempted to have sex, so that her response of freezing up and dissociating was immediately triggered the moment she made eye contact during intimacy.

One way to begin working with this kind of rigid stimulus-response trance phenomenon is by creating new associations to the dreaded stimulus. You interrupt the pattern, in essence, simply by expanding the client's associative frames of reference in regard to the sensitive area. For example:

> "And, which eye looks more threatening. . .the left or the right? Which eye looks more friendly. . .the left or the right? And I probably do not have to tell you what is left for you might not be what is right for you, or what is right for you might not be what is left for you."

Here I am attempting to differentiate her focus of attention on one eye and expand it to include two eyes. Later I'll expand it to include the two eyes, the nose and mouth—all of which continues to differentiate the trigger of the left eye. Any differentiations or reassociations in the trigger alter the response pattern. (See Chapter 18, "Differentiating and Reassociating the Trigger.")

I am often asked if this type of reassociating is the same as the Ericksonian technique of reframing. It is not. In reframing, the experience itself remains the same; what changes is the context within which it is held. For example, a spiritually oriented person going through a traumatic life situation might describe his experience by saying, "I'm learning a lot of lessons right now." A more psychologically oriented person would say, "I'm growing a lot." When I lived in India, some of us at the monastery would chuckle when reading letters from similarly seeking friends, who would write about how much they were "growing." We would say, "god, they must really be in pain!" The experience of a traumatic life situation remains the same; only its label or frame is changed.

In reassociation, by contrast, you create completely new associations that carry multiple meanings and interrupt the stimulus-response prototype. The stimulus called "men" no longer elicits the response called "fear" because you have created new stimuli and new associations. By creating these new associations, the pattern can no longer occur one-on-one; you have already broadened it to one-on-ten: ". . .And you can notice that Uncle Henry actually has two eyes. . .and a mouth. . .and two cheeks. . .and a nose. . .not to mention a forehead. . .a chin. . .and two temples."

Retrieving Resources. Whenever age regression emerges in a client, you can use it to retrieve inner resources. Indeed, once the fixed nature of the Deep Trance Phenomenon of age regression is altered via reassociation, developmental resources long suppressed will usually "float" to surface. These resources are often comprised of those cherished but squashed childhood qualities of openness, vulnerability, and the free expression of emotion.

I worked with a client who complained that he was unable to be intimate. Every time he entered a relationship with a woman, it ended after only a few months with a frustrated lament from his partner to the effect of, "You're completely invulnerable! I can't touch you. You're walled off, in a safe and distant zone." When I asked him to recreate that state of invulnerability while breathing and looking at me, he gradually age-regressed in his speech and began acting out what appeared to be a scene from his childhood. In this re-creation, he was a child of three, trying to crawl onto his mother's lap and cuddle. She kept telling him to get away and leave her alone. This type of incident was repeated often enough that his response to it become automatic. To defend against his mother's rebuff, he "shut down," became hard and cold, walling himself off from experiencing this event with his mother. What is crucial to understand is that if he lets go of the wall in present time, he will experience the pain of rejection which the wall is defending him against feeling.

Decades later, this man is still bringing his mother with him into each and every encounter he has with women. And each time, when confronted with the possibility of an emotionally intimate exchange, he age-regresses into his walled-off area by tightening his muscles, holding his breath, and freezing up. This age-regressed trance has been enacted and re-enacted hundreds of times with the same, astounding precision. That is why once this particular trance phenomenon is altered (via reassociation or differentiation, which we'll discuss later), those developmental resources that were suppressed by the child's defensive trance will become available to the adult in present time.

Tapping on the door of the fixed trance sets in motion a fail-safe, no-lose therapeutic process, because sooner or later, you're going to encounter resources—provided you know how to recognize them. *Any* resisted experience is a potential resource. And, since Deep Trance Phenomena are the "guardians" of a multitude of resisted experiences, they are a veritable storehouse of resources. Any experience can be a resource.

I have been challenged on this point. *Everything is a resource?*, comes the incredulous question. In my experience, the answer is yes. Anger is a resource, depression is a resource, not knowing is a resource, even "blah-ness" is a resource. I had a client who as a child had never been allowed "to just be blah." Her parents were, as she described them, "very zippity-do-dah"—always *up*, always energized and emoting about something. As an adult, she had a problem with chronic, mild depression—she seemed forever stuck in (age regressed to) the dreaded blah feeling. She needed to fully experience the forbidden state free of judgement, solely from the position of the witness. For her as an adult, the experience of feeling blah *without judgment* was wonderful. Instead of it turning into a lingering depression, she experienced her blah-ness as a time just for herself when she had complete permission to just *be*. It is a grand paradox: as long as you evaluate blah-ness as being something bad you shouldn't experience, you're constantly going to resist it—which, in turn, keeps the blah-ness ever-present.

Another case example that illustrates the axiom that everything is a resource involved a man for whom the response of "I don't know" became a liberating experience. This man was obsessed with a sensation of pain in his right teste, for which no organic cause had been found. By the time he came to see me, his entire life virtually revolved around his awareness of this pain. It was not acute, but he was chronically distraught that no name or cause could be attached to explain it. He kept saying over and over, "I just have to know what's causing it." It wasn't enough that several doctors had assured him there was nothing organically wrong.

I asked him to breathe and look at me as he focused on his symptom. He began to describe it, and with each adjective, I asked him to exaggerate the sensation a little bit more. After a few minutes, it became apparent that he had age regressed. Suddenly, he was six months old and lying in a crib crying. I continued to have him "breathe and look at me" as he re-experienced the infant's distress. Then he began saying over and over, "I don't know. . .I don't know. . .I don't know." By this time, the baby was kicking and screaming, throwing off his blankets. The adults kept trying to comfort him by saying, "It's alright." But this simply prevented him from experiencing the frustration of, "I don't know."

As he grew older, this resistance to "I don't know" was intensified when his father was institutionalized with a nervous breakdown. Being the oldest, his mother repeatedly exhorted him to *know*. Having to know became an opposing identity to "I don't know." He so resisted *not knowing* that he received two Ph.Ds. The problem was that both states or identities were age-regressed states. The "I-have-to-know" state tried to overcompensate for the "I-don't-know state." The pain in his teste began to subside upon acknowledging the resource of a willingness to experience "I don't know." As homework, I suggested he give himself permission to *not* have all the answers—to say simply, "I don't know."

When this client returned the following week, he was a geyser of insights and connections. We had not discussed the regression experience in the session, as I did not want him undoing it with his mind. Over the past week, however, countless associations had floated to the surface as he connected to very early experiences where, as he put it: "I had to know how to hold a bottle, I had to know how to crawl, I had to know how to walk, I had to know how to recognize Mommy and Daddy. I had to know how to be a man when my father was institutionalized. It feels like I was having to show everything I knew from the time I was an infant."

As an infant, this client had not been allowed to have the

experience of "I don't know." Repression of this perfectly valid I-don't-know response throughout his life had created a cycle of pressure, strain, stress, and, finally, physical symptomatology. When "I don't know" emerged in his trance work, I recognized it immediately as a key resource. In this next session we focused solely on the feeling of "I don't know." As usual, I asked him to breathe and look at me while he experienced the deliciousness (his word) of *not knowing* in a multitude of contexts. To reinforce this work, and help integrate it into his real life, I gave him a homework assignment in which, five times a day, he was to answer a question with the words, "I don't know," and simply observe how it felt.

Axiom: *Everything can be a resource.*

Injecting Trauma with Resources. In my view, our ability to age-regress should never be used to *induce* the re-experience of a trauma. Rather, when the client brings in age regression as the main Deep Trance Phenomenon underlying her symptom, you can use it, in essence, to restructure the past trauma by adding all the resources accumulated over a lifetime of coping. It is not unlike the medical technique of skin grafting, in which a minuscule patch of healthy skin cells is "harvested" and placed over the damaged tissue: almost instantaneously, the blood vessels underneath the injured area begin to grow up toward the graft to integrate it. So it can be with damaged psyches.

In making use of a spontaneous age regression, it is important to note that I do not give suggestions to re-experience a past trauma directly. Instead, I hold the person in present time and establish myself as the context via eye contact while he or she retrieves the experience. This method accomplishes two important tasks: *it brings accumulated resources into the trauma equation*, and *the trauma is recontextualized in present time*. Let's take a brief look at each of these.

It is safe to assume that any adult client who comes to you with a major childhood trauma has a well-developed storehouse of resources that has allowed her/him to survive. The usual approach to reliving trauma as a means of healing it is to have the client regress and relive the experience as it occurred in past time. The problem is, *this* is *present time*, and the client is not the same person as the child. I do not want to discount a lifetime of experience in creating resources to deal with the trauma; I want the client to bring these resources with her when she re-encounters that terrible time.

The second benefit of this particular approach to reliving trauma is that the client takes the therapist with her. The directive, "Breathe and look at me," helps the client take the present (embodied in the therapist) with her, back to the time of the trauma—which, in essence, changes the context in which it is re-experienced. Now she has two strong foundations of resources with which to re-experience the trauma: the foundation of accumulated resources forged over a lifetime of coping; and the foundation of present reality, with all its larger contexts.

Let me divert here for a moment to elaborate a technique I developed for diffusing transference and projection when dealing, in particular, with molestation traumas. As a male therapist working with women reliving such traumas, I realized that the potential for my being viewed as the perpetrator at some point or other in the trance process was quite high. To deflect that development, I would direct the client to select a particular feature about me that would be associated with a clear recognition of who I was and when it was. For example:

> "I'd like you to look at me now and pick out something—
> it might be my beard, it might be my glasses, it might be the
> rings on my fingers. And every time you look at that, you
> will know that my name is Stephen and it is 1989."

Whenever the client's expressions began to indicate fusion with me as the perpetrator, I would say, "And as you continue to look at my glasses (or wherever), you know that I am Stephen, and that it is 1989. . . . And what is your experience like right now?" To return to the skin-graft metaphor, the therapist together with the client's inner resources represent the graft of healthy tissue being repositioned over the traumatized areas of the psyche. You have to keep the graft in position—you have to keep the client in present time—in order for deep healing to occur.

Treatment of Age Regression

Rather than adhering to a strict (and often arbitrary) division between therapist and client, I have chosen to tread both arenas. The underlying assumption is that there isn't really any fundamental difference between a person being called "therapist" and a person being called "client." Therefore, a therapeutic technology geared for use by the individual can be meaningful for both.

In each of the chapters dealing with specific Deep Trance Phenomena, a concluding section on Treatment will provide suggestions for the individual to use in working *within* on his or her own trances, or with others' trances.

Now, let's explore various approaches for age regression.

Suggestion I: Witnessing and Expanding the Age-Regressed Trance

First, begin to learn to identify when you are slipping into an age-regressed state in your daily life. Perhaps you are having a disagreement with your spouse and you feel a sense of being out-of-control coming over you; perhaps you have been reprimanded on the job and you are gripped with the impulse to throw a temper tantrum. Or perhaps it is something far more subtle: like, during an interaction with a colleague, you find yourself using various types of manipulative behaviors to win his/her favor. Whatever the particular outer circumstances, and whatever the particular shades and shapes of your individual age regression experience, begin to witness when it occurs.

(1) If possible, take some time out for yourself. If you are at work, take your break in a quiet area where, ideally, you can lie down. Let yourself go deeply into the sensations you are experiencing, and as you are doing so, witness them. The simple act of witnessing expands the experience, expands *you*, for you are no longer totally identified with it; part of you is observing. The circumference of your self has expanded to incorporate the activity of witnessing.

(2) Now you are in two simultaneous states: the age-regressed state of the pouting child (or whatever), and the state of the observing witness. Notice, next, if there are any resources, feelings, thoughts, or actions that might be of help to the part of you that is age-regressed. For example, perhaps it would help to give the age-regressed part certain messages or resources. Talk to it, like you would talk to a living child, telling it what it needs to hear.

(3) Now allow all these new resources to merge and join with

the age-regressed part so that they become an organic whole. As they become integrated—as you embrace the child, merge with the child, become the child—you are bringing your age-regressed inner child into present time.

Now your current behavior is no longer context-independent. In a sense, you have time-traveled: You have brought the age-regressed parts of your self into the context of the present moment. Your attention is no longer narrowed and fixated in the trance state and can now expand and respond fully.

Suggestion II: Revisioning Trauma

Erickson's ingenious case of the "February Man" (Erickson & Rossi, 1989) contains the prototype for this approach to healing trauma. As the February Man, Erickson "visited" his client during several age-regressed sessions, during which her various traumas were re-experienced in the context of the added wisdom, insight, and support provided by this figure of the wise old man. In the approach described below, the client recreates several states of being that now co-exist in relation to the trauma. Each state of being arises entirely within the client: the child prior to the trauma (if the trauma occurred when the child was 6, then this child is 5), the child in the trauma, the adult, and the person who has successfully resolved the trauma in present time (via pseudo-orientation in time). We now have four different states of being:

State I: The child prior to the trauma
State II: The child in the trauma
State III: The adult in present time
State IV: The adult who has used the Deep Trance Phenom-
              enon of pseudo-orientation in time to resolve the
              trauma.

There is an obvious benefit to this particular slant, which is that it reduces if not eliminates the tendency of the client to project his/her strengths and resources onto the therapist. Erickson's February Man approach is more open to such projection—especially when attempted by those of us less skilled clinically than Erickson.

The steps to this approach are as follows:

(1) See the child *prior to* the traumatic event.

(2) See the child as an *older person* with the situation handled or resolved.

(3) Have the *older person* in Step 2 join the *child* in Step 1 to look into future events, knowing that they will occur. The older person gives suggestions that counter those that were part of the trauma. (For example, in a molest case, the older person might counsel the child with the injunctions, "All men aren't like this...You can trust a lot of men, you just can't trust this one...Be careful of certain types of men, but feel free to feel safe with the right ones...")

(4) Now the *older person* and the *child* plan what to do, given the upcoming trauma that is about to occur. For example, they consider what might be helpful to remember or understand as the event unfolds.

(5) After the new course of action is determined, have the three parts merge: the *child* prior to the trauma, vulnerable and without resources...merges with the *older person* who has handled the trauma...which merges with the *child who now re-experiences the trauma with the added support and help of all the accumulated resources of the adult in present time.* All three coalesce, as they experience being with the new resources, ideas, plans, and so forth.

(6) Now bring all parts into present time to experience integration and resolution.

For example, a child is molested at age 6. The adult comes to therapy at age 26 around this issue.

Step I: Have the 26-year-old go into the future to a place where the trauma is handled.

Step II: Have the 26-year-old go to a place prior to the occurrence of the trauma.

Step III: Bring together the person in Step I with the person in Step II and look forward to the event that has not happened, knowing that it will happen.

Step IV: Have the age-progressed person give advice on how to handle the upcoming trauma.

Step V: Have the child prior to the trauma, the traumatized child, the adult in present time, and the age-progressed person all merge.

To vary the client's experience of the Deep Trance Phenomenon is to depotentiate the strength of the presenting symptom or problem. I have already discussed how my approach to altering the Deep Trance Phenomenon underlying symptomatology differs from Erickson's technique of pattern interruption in which he used induced therapeutic trance states to interrupt or block the occurrence of the symptom.

8

Age Progression:
Pseudo-Orientation
In Time

We TIME-TRAVEL in many ways. Age *regression*, as we just saw, is one way; age *progression* is another. More often called *pseudo-orientation in time*, the purpose of this Deep Trance Phenomenon is projection of oneself into the future when an imagined, more pleasant environment protects us or distracts us from the distressing, ongoing interactions of the present. Like all Deep Trance Phenomena, pseudo-orientation in time is created by a series of *inter*personal interactions during childhood that threaten one's psycho-emotional survival. By creating a future free of the immediate conflicts and injuries, the child helps himself/ herself get through the day. An *intra*personal trance response is thus created over time via repeated use so that it begins to function automatically; conscious intentionality is no longer necessary to initiate the trance defense.

We all use pseudo-orientation in time to envision our futures in much brighter colors than are present moments appear. Who hasn't toyed with a fantasy of being rich and famous, living on the ocean-front, with a scintillating career and dazzling spouse?

I have quite clear memories of my series of fantasies, spanning childhood through teenage years, in which I happily re-oriented myself to a time in the future when. . . . I was a baseball star, but then I was confronted by the harsh reality of not being good at it. . . .Football stardom crumbled when I realized my 5'7" frame would never make it through a game . . . . Rock-n'-roll stardom fizzled underneath the weight of absolutely no musical aptitude whatsoever. . . .and my passion to become a lawyer, which constellated while watching the movie, *Inherit the Wind*, slowly waned as Clarence Darrow's inspiring books butted up against the drudgery of law school.

Whenever we engage in these kinds of fantasies, we are in a Deep Trance Phenomenon—which is no problem in and of itself. It only becomes a problem when it impedes our ability to deal with current issues. For example, if my entire childhood, adolescence, and teenage years had been consumed by these fantasies, to the point where I had isolated myself from real-life experience, I would certainly have suffered a significant developmental lack.

In adulthood, we continue to use pseudo-orientation in time to transport us forward to our dreams, wishes, and desires. Again, this can be fine when it is circumscribed by a solid grounding in ongoing reality. Flights of fantasy in which we creatively project our awareness into the future are one thing; *flights* of fantasy in which we are truly (but unknowingly) *fleeing* from our life in the present is another matter altogether. Pseudo-orientation in time removes interpersonal feedback by removing the loop between self and other, leaving only the self-to-self trance.

Perhaps the most salient, contemporary example of how an adult can use pseudo-orientation in time symptomatically is the classic fantasy of the struggling co-dependent person who spends his life imagining what it will be like when his father (or mother, brother, wife) finally *changes* and gives him what he wants. Or there is the example of the addict who obsessively fantasizes about how great things will be once he handles his addiction. *The fantasy of the future is thus used as a means of resisting what is actually being experienced in the present.*

Another example: If I continually imagine myself in an incredibly wonderful relationship, I might be resisting my current experience of either not being in any kind of a relationship, or being in an dissatisfying one. The fantasy is a deceptive cloak; it keeps me content enough to *not* make any significant changes in my life—floating, as it were, a few feet above actual lived experience. "In the clouds" is an apt description of the net result of this particular use of pseudo-orientation in time.

Another example: I know a woman who is 35 years old and has lived in Salt Lake City, Utah, for most of her life. She continues to harbor a very vivid fantasy about becoming an actress. In fact, she told me that she thinks about this all the time; she can actually "see herself" in Hollywood in the "near future." Yet, she does not move to Los Angeles where she would at least stand a chance of entering the field; and she does not even take acting lessons in Salt Lake City. This woman is creating an obsessional looping that has absolutely no feedback in present reality, made possible by the altered state of pseudo-orientation in time.

These examples illustrate how the Deep Trance Phenomenon of pseudo-orientation in time, originally formed in childhood, gains autonomous functioning over the years. When first used by the child as a buffer for discomfort or threat, the trance was "context dependent": its emergence depended on particular, formative events that "triggered" the protective response. As this pattern was reinforced, it was gradually put on automatic—a behaviorist would say that the response became "generalized" and "habituated." It is now context *independent*, adrift from its original causative source (unwanted feelings in the body). The specific allure of pseudo-orientation in time is its link with childhood flights of fantasy, where the possibility of magical solutions still glitters in a bittersweet way. This power to leave real life and enter another realm where we finally feel we have control becomes addictive. In this way, an adult can become chronically enmeshed in an internal fantasy life (an intrapersonal trance) about the future rather than experiencing the ongoing ebb and flow of the *now*.

Varieties of Pseudo-Orientation in Time

Posthypnotic Suggestions. When I saw myself as a football star, or a brilliant lawyer, or a baseball star, I was using predominantly visual imagery to construct the inner pictures. Movie-like sequences unfolded as if there were a projector sitting inside my mind. Another form of pseudo-orientation in time makes use of post-hypnotic suggestions to inject the fantasy with specific directives or messages—whatever is most needed by the psyche.

I worked with a woman, for example, who kept having involuntary fantasies which were so real to her that they were no longer fantasies—they were fact. Beings from another dimension were telling her that she was going to be the next Christ. She was very anxiety-ridden about this, feeling unprepared for such a task. Let me say, first, that I don't automatically label someone as psychotic if they report extraordinary experiences, nor do I assume that such experiences are imaginary. However, I had little doubt about this woman; her personal pathology was quite clearly apparent.

The evolution of her other-dimensional beings began in childhood when, as primary caretaker of her sick father while her mother worked to support them, she was isolated from normal childhood friendships. She coped with her barren social life by creating imaginary friends who began giving her very specific messages such as: "One day, you'll be beautiful and famous". . . ."One day, you'll have a two-story house, two kids, a husband and a maid". . . ."One day, your father will tell you how wonderful you are, and how he couldn't get along without you."

As a young adult, she married a man who was extremely needy and very demanding. She found herself, once again, in a dreary role as caretaker where her own dreams and desires languished, just as they had throughout her childhood. Her "visitations" began after five years of marriage, at a very low point in her life. The beings told her to persevere; her time would come when she would be recognized and heralded as the world's Savior.

Whether Christ fantasies or Beatles fantasies populate your inner life, the problem of "re-entry" inevitably arises: How do you get back into the real world? How do you get back into your body? Once this Deep Trance Phenomenon has been put on automatic, there is no feedback loop in the present-day interpersonal context. In essence, we remain suspended in a mental plane of time-travel, with only varying degrees of "rootedness" to the three-dimensional world of physical life.

Age Regression. Often, pseudo-orientation in time also involves the Deep Trance Phenomenon of age regression. Put more simply, we all have a tendency to look back at the past and project it into the future. The past state becomes frozen in time, remains as a context for the present, and is also projected into the future. Chronic anxiety in the adult, which is a response to frozen traumas of the past, requires the Deep Trance Phenomenon of pseudo-orientation in time if it is to remain *chronic*. In this state, there really is no sense of time as we commonly experience it; the linear quality of forward motion is completely lacking. A blanket, negative association to the future is created and sustained out of the traumas of the past—with the help of the Deep Trance Phenomena.

The particular combination of pseudo-orientation in time and age regression is probably at the basis of about three-quarters of the symptomatology you'll encounter—both in yourself and in your clients. It is also an important example of how the various Deep Trance Phenomenon cluster, interweave, and interact to create an effective defense for the individual.

Case Example

I worked with a woman whose presenting problem was projectile vomiting. She had just finished a rigorous training program in biology and was working for a firm. Her symptom suggested that she was projecting catastrophe into the future in some way that she could not stomach. Before making that assumption, however, I wanted her to show me which Deep Trance Phenomena *she* was using to create her symptom.

I began by asking her to find the position her body is in when the vomiting starts, and to "continue to breathe and look at me." Soon she murmured, "I'm losing ground. . . .I'm losing ground." She quickly began to age regress, as evidenced by a change in body posture and facial expression. As I watched her I spontaneously began to talk to the little girl I was beginning to perceive before me, talking about "little girls who had to take care of themselves and how they were afraid to let go." I also addressed the concerned adult who was "losing ground."

The issue here is that once a frozen trauma is held and projected into the future, the feedback loop of the body is replaced by the trance of pseudo-orientation in time. This particular technique helps the client to get back in touch with his or her body, which has been forsaken in favor of the Deep Trance Phenomenon.

Case Example

A woman came to see me because she was experiencing acute anxiety from the fact that her divorce would be final in the next two weeks and "she would lose everything." Her statement of the problem was enough to tell me that her primary trance symptom was pseudo-orientation in time: projecting a catastrophic outcome in the future and experiencing it in present time. I began to work with this trance by asking her to continue to re-create it for me in as much detail as possible, beginning with her body posture.

Slowly, as she recited the negative suggestions she saw as descriptive of her future, her shoulders slumped forward, her knees drew in rigidly, she clasped her hands tightly together, and fixed her eyes on the ground. I asked her to "breathe and look at me" as she continued, so she lifted her eyes, leaving her chin and head hanging in a downward position. In a faint, weak voice she began muttering, "He's going to get the house. . . .He's going to get the savings account. . . .He's going to get the certificate accounts. . . .He's going to get the furniture."

I took over her internal dialogue by repeating her statements and asking her to repeat them also.* In an earlier chapter, we saw how intensifying the dynamic that creates the symptomatology paradoxically helps the person move out of it into an expanded state. This patient proceeded to demonstrate this Ericksonian principle of "the symptom is the cure" perfectly: After several minutes of repeating her negative self-suggestions, she grew quiet and her body posture "melted" and softened. I asked her what she was

---

*In the hypnosis work of this example, I am "taking over" the trance so that the client no longer has to do it. In recent years other therapists have adopted the approach of "taking over" the client's resistance: for example, in the Feldenkrais Method of body work, in Ron Kurtz's Hakomi therapy and, more recently, in the process-oriented therapy of Arnold Mindell. This take-over approach was also utilized in the psychodrama methods of the mid-1970s in which group members were invited to "play the part" of the voices that were active within a client's mind. In each form of therapy, clients no longer had to "do" their voices or resistances, which freed them to explore themselves in a different way. In psychodrama, gestalt therapy, as well as the process-oriented therapy of Arnold Mindell, clients are asked to *exaggerate* their experience, which helps them to own, incorporate, and integrate disowned parts of themselves.

experiencing and after a deep sigh she responded, "I can see the light at the end of the tunnel." From my perspective, "taking over" the client's self-induced trance (by repeating the statements out loud) takes over the conscious mind and allows the resources ("the light at the end of the tunnel") to emerge.

I pursued her metaphorical description, associating it verbally with the pending divorce settlement and adding progressive suggestions that created a two-week time-frame. The two weeks were not experienced day by day but as an undifferentiated mass of time that was emotionally and psychologically overwhelming. In such situations, I create a time-period as well as define clear, signposted steps to mark progress. Erickson has often commented that we tend to overlook our successes; much of what he did was to resurrect these successes and present them back to the patient so that he or she could appreciate and enjoy each step along the way.

In this case, I understood the client's statement about light at the end of the tunnel to verify her unconscious perception of a favorable outcome, and then took her back and forth, across a time-period of 14 days and across a latticework of 14 steps. Each day was a step toward the light at the end of the tunnel—something like the "twelve days of Christmas" theme—and held a particular accomplishment for her. I kept the suggestions very general so that her own unconscious resources could fill in the specifics.

I also had her looking back at the 14 days, the 14 steps, from the perspective of *having already arrived* at the light at the end of the tunnel. I used suggestions that remained general to review each step's unique point and marveling at how all the steps coalesced into such a radiant, unified light.

I let the suggestions "set" in silence for a few minutes and then asked her what she was feeling. She said, "I feel like a butterfly." I took her butterfly metaphor as another resource and utilized it in suggestions such as: "How nice it is to know you can be at step 14 and look back at step 11...and step 7...and even steps 3 and 1." For quite a while she experienced herself in trance flying back and forth, exploring each one of the steps.

My most salient objective with this client was to help her use her own trance choice of pseudo-orientation in time to create a pleasant future. I also wanted her to the return to the present, keeping all the wonderful feelings of freedom she had experienced as a butterfly.

I used the metaphor of the butterfly, which *she* had given me, to facilitate her ease in moving back and forth in time from the perspective of the free butterfly rather than the anxiety-ridden woman.

Another client came to me with the fear of not being able to make his mortgage payments six months in the future. He was running a "What if" scenario: *What if* I lose my job. . . . *What if* I get sick. Since he was demonstrating pseudo-orientation in time as his problem, that is what I worked with. In trance I began talking about when I was a small boy, I would lie in the grass and look at clouds, imagining devil-like faces (this was a metaphor for the client's pseudo-orientation in time as an undifferentiated mass in the future). I then suggested that he might also see cowboys, horses, and pots of gold in the clouds. As I offered differentiations to his Deep Trance Phenomenon, his rigid trance shifted and expanded to incorporate the new elements and alleviate his anxiety.

Treatment of Pseudo-Orientation in Time

I. *Planning Backwards.* I first saw this approach demonstrated by Carol and Stephen Lankton. Have your client (or yourself) experience a time in the future when the problem is already resolved. Carefully plan how to move back from the future vantage point where the problem is resolved to the present where the problem remains. Do this by identifying a resource in the form of a symbol (like the butterfly), a new perspective (such as phantom limb *pleasure*—see below), an image (the light at the end of the tunnel), a word, feeling, or sensation. Experience it *right now*.

For example, a client came to me who was feeling extremely anxious and agitated about passing her oral examination for her Ph.D. Using her own trance of pseudo-orientation in time, I guided her to a time in the future when she had received her doctorate and was feeling relieved. Next I asked her to bring back that deep sense of relief into the present in the form of a resource. She saw an image of a dove and heard the word *accomplishment*, which she was encouraged to experience *right now*.

II. *Reversing Catastrophic Outcomes.* Erickson's ingenious

statement to an amputee patient, "Since you have phantom limb *pain*, why not have phantom limb *pleasure*?", becomes the foundation for this next technique. Any time your client expresses what appears to be a negative inevitability, look for its opposite, as Erickson did. If a client can torment herself by imagining a catastrophic outcome to her situation, she can also delight herself by imagining a pleasant outcome.

You can add gradations to this method, as I did above with the clouds, so that it does not sound simplistic; these gradations mix and blend the catastrophic outcome with the pleasant outcome rather than offering one as the alternative to the other. I have often used a personal example to communicate this concept while working hypnotically with the client:

"When I was a little boy, I used to lie down on the grass and look up at clouds. I would watch the clouds form all these different faces and shapes and colors. First, there would be a very, very ugly face—like a fierce devil. And I'd watch the ugly, terrible face/cloud, transfixed. Then I'd shake my head and refocus my eyes and see big, fluffy, beautiful clouds that held a rainbow, a unicorn, a pot of gold. Then I'd blink and the devil's face would be back, and at the same time, those fluffy beautiful shapes would begin to shift and float and change and there would be a cowboy, or maybe it was a cowgirl, in the center."

Here, I am taking the Deep Trance Phenomenon of pseudo-orientation in time, which is a formless mass at the basis of the client's fear of the future, and differentiating it into comprehensible portions. I identify the "bad" in the form of a menacing face, and then I add a little of the "good" in the form of a rainbow, a unicorn, a pot of gold. I intersperse options, beginning with the client's most anxious reality, and then alternate with the positive reality. In a sense, I am juggling both realities at once: terrible, excellent, terrible, excellent, terrible, excellent—until the sharp lines of both realities begin to blend and blur. To use an artistic analogy, the primary colors of the two realities have been intermixed to produce a new array of softer hues and tones. What this means clinically is that the Deep Trance Phenomenon that is creating the client's symptom has been altered—which means the symptom itself has been altered.

The future can be experienced in the present, either automatically through the Deep Trance Phenomenon of pseudo-orientation in time, or consciously, by choosing to project one's awareness into the future. When a fear of negative outcomes is at the core of the client's presenting problem, you know that the client has created a trance of pseudo-orientation in time and put it on automatic. By differentiating the mass or block of time called "future" into small steps, while holding the desired outcome in the present, the client can create and experience the desired outcome *now*.

9

Dissociation

W HEN I FIRST watched the movie *Sybil* two decades ago, I was completely mystified by what I saw: a woman being transformed *within herself* from one personality to another. Complete changes in appearance, voice, posture, and expression accompanied each shift into another personality—as did a total amnesia for the experience. I found it difficult to fathom how so many aspects of one person's self could split off so completely and comprehensively!

After having a few opportunities to work with multiple personalities, I began to appreciate the incredible versatility of the phenomenon. The mind's extraordinary ability to survive and protect itself was demonstrated to me by a client, a woman, who had been so severely sexually abused that she had dissociated from the experience, surrounded it in amnesia, and created a boy personality. So effective was this personality that she did not begin her menstrual cycle until she was 22 years old.

Another amazing aspect of multiple personality is that each personality not only acts autonomously, but lives its own life within the context of only one body. So, for the "boy" personality in the woman to become aware would require an insight or understanding of *why* and *what* had happened to create such a powerful survival mechanism or trance.

Today I look at the phenomenon called multiple personality and view it as part of the continuum of trances "normal" people live. It is certainly more dramatic than what most of us experience, and for that reason serves as a template of Deep Trance Phenomena potentialities. Multiple personality is made possible by a multifaceted network of just such phenomena—clusters of trance states are utilized to synthesize and apportion the various personalities.

Perhaps the most dominant trance "ingredient" of multiple personality is dissociation, which is used to demarcate, as it were, portions of the person's psyche into separate units. So thoroughly can the dissociation be affected that the person's physical body actually undergoes major and measurable changes as the personalities come and go: shoe sizes change, eye colors vacillate, allergic responses appear in one personality but not in the others, and so on.

Multiple personality provides us with an awesome portrait of the Deep Trance Phenomenon of dissociation at its most potent and exotic. Many incest survivors, while not developing multiple personalities, used dissociation to survive as children. Problems arise when years after the trauma, this effective skill or resource no longer fits the context and becomes autonomous, operating outside of the person's control. Less dramatic versions of dissociation are experienced by most adults on a daily basis: we "space out" or "move far away" in situations that threaten or stress us.

Erickson (1952/1980) regarded dissociation as a key ingredient of therapeutic trance, in which healing occurred via the dissociation of conscious and unconscious processes: "Deep hypnosis is that level of hypnosis that permits the subject to function adequately and directly at an unconscious level of awareness without interference from the conscious mind" (p. 146).

For Erickson and Rossi (1979), trance also facilitates the dissociation of a person's learned limitations from his/her untapped resources and mental associations, thus freeing these for problem-solving.

By contrast, in my concept of the trance/no-trance continuum discussed earlier, dissociation from one part of the psyche and attachment to another is not the goal. Rather, the goal is an equal and fluid relationship among all the psyche's currents and rivulets. I do not evoke dissociation as a means of creating the experience of therapeutic trance (although there are exceptions, which I will discuss below). Instead, the client's *presentation of dissociation* as the trance state underlying his/her problem or symptom would be utilized and altered as the means of treatment. Like all Deep Trance Phenomena, dissociation is originally created by a series of interpersonal interactions in a given context to support, maintain, and protect the child from an environment that is experienced as threatening. The child learns to cope with the sensation of threat by "taking off," "spacing out," "floating to the top of the ceiling," "going somewhere else."

Dissociation can be experienced in three modalities:

(1) dissociation from an internal feeling, sensation, or emotion;
(2) dissociation from a part of the body (genitals, limbs, voice, muscles, etc.);
(3) dissociation from external stimuli.

Dissociation from an Internal State. Most of us have particular emotions or states-of-being we are extremely unwilling to experience: sadness, anger, fear, enthusiasm, passivity, and so on. Usually, these aversions were established via childhood experiences in which parents, for one reason or another, disallowed a particular response in the child. I had one client, for example, who was terrified of feeling sad. As a child, his parents' typical response to him was, "Joseph, now smile." The parents were extremely over-identified with their only son and could not tolerate any signs of discomfort from him. "Joseph, now smile," became an oppressive injunction in the child's life that had endured into adulthood.

Another client was physically beaten by her father, whose violence would increase if she showed any signs of experiencing pain. To survive, she learned how to effectively dissociate from the pain and sadness. When she began therapy 25 years later, she was literally unable to feel; indeed, she did not know what a "feeling" was. Although this client demonstrated an extreme use of dissociation, most of us dissociate mildly from anger or other unwanted emotions by saying, "I'm not myself today," or "I don't know what came over me," or "That wasn't me, it was the alcohol."

Dissociation from a Body Part. This form of dissociation is much more common than it might sound. Dissociation is an ongoing trance state that is part of the way in which the person "lives" in his/

her body. It is important to recognize that dissociation of body parts is really quite common. I had a client who experienced his mouth as being separate from himself. He did not experience the words his mouth produced as coming from within—from the Self. It was all "lip-service," as he put it. In other words, he was dissociating from himself and his feelings to produce the "appropriate" communication—what his parents wanted to hear. To produce these words, he dissociated from his own mouth, which resulted in the feeling that his mouth was acting autonomously.

Sexual dysfunction generally involves dissociation from the genital area. In cases of impotence or premature ejaculation, the penis is dissociated from the rest of the man's body; in Gestalt terms, the figure (penis) is separated from the ground (body). Indeed, even when male genitals do "function" adequately, we are often dissociated from them. Robin Williams has used his comedic genius to highlight the tendency men have to give names to their penises—Fred, Marlin, Dick, Macko, Mister Happy—as if they were something entirely separate from the men themselves.

The same dynamic operates in pre-orgasmic women: vaginal response (figure) is dissociated from the rest of the woman's body (ground).

Another common example of this type of dissociation from a part of the body is the migraine headache. You don't have a migraine in your foot, or in your back, or in your stomach; it is isolated (dissociated) from the rest of the body. In Chapter 6 I presented several "Expanded Contexts of Healing," beginning with "Expanding the Context to Include the Body." That technique is pertinent in this area of physical/psychosomatic dysfunction. For example, when working with migraine, you begin by spreading the sensation of a headache throughout the entire body so that it becomes a totally unified experience:

"Now as you feel the sensations of headache in your eyes or ears or just the top of your head, it can. . .become easy to notice the sensations moving to include your nose, which knows how you can. . .experience the sensations, vibrations, permutations, or combinations of sensations in your chest."

Eventually, the background or body is included in the experience and connects the head (foreground) to it, providing a different experience of expanded context.

Similarly, in cases of sexual dysfunction, I begin by teaching the person to allow the sexual sensations throughout the body so that they are no longer isolated (dissociated) in one small region. Here, again, we are reuniting the figure with the ground. In bioenergetic terms, "streaming" occurs whereby sensations are moving throughout the body. Earlier roots for this technique can be found in the practices of Tantric yoga, where sexual sensations are gathered and spread throughout the body rather than being dissipated through orgasm in one localized area.

One way of working with this dynamic is by using suggestion to expand the context of the person's experience to include the entire body, as suggested in Chapter 6.

Erickson made use of his personal experiences with dissociation that arose from his bouts with polio as an experiential foundation for suggesting dissociation of various body parts as he worked with subjects in trance. Typically, he used the patient's hypnotic response of dissociation as a means of "ratifying" the trance: if the patient could no longer feel his feet on the ground, obviously something other than ordinary consciousness was afoot.

Since I begin from the assumption that the person is already in trance, I do not need to suggest or induce it. Rather, I observe the client's behavior and, if I see that there is a body dissociation going on, I will then begin to work with it.

Dissociation from External Stimuli. When the outer world becomes too threatening or assaultive, the child learns to "leave" it in the only way he can—by dissociating from it. He may simply "space out" into a somnambulistic trance state, or he may actively imagine himself in some other location. Either way, his first action is to dissociate his psycho-emotional presence from the immediate physical environment. To continue our Gestalt terminology, the figure of the child is dissociated from the ground of the external environment.

The concept of dissociation can be used very liberally. Whenever a client is not experiencing his own inner resources, for example, that means he is dissociated from those resources. If the client is experiencing age regression, it means she is dissociated from present time; if she is experiencing pseudo-orientation in time, she is dissociated from present time. In fact, the presence of any Deep Trance Phenomenon means that the person is dissociated in a significant way from some part of the internal or external environment.

Developing Oppositional Trances

One way of working with entrenched trance patterns is to help the person experience an oppositional trance. For example, if a client habitually uses dissociation as a means of responding to his world, you can introduce him to its opposite: over-identification. You might ask him to re-create his dissociative state and, once he is in a deep trance, begin to suggest that he look at and feel and sense the situation he is in, and that he begin to totally merge with it, become it, identify with it. And so on.

Conversely, an over-identified client would begin by allowing herself to fully experience the over-identification, and then gradually begin to witness it more and more and more, until she is watching it from a distance—dissociation.

This approach is not as naturalistic as the main one of simply utilizing and altering the trance presented by clients; here, I am actually giving direct suggestions for them to experience something else. This is the only context in which I actively suggest trance states to clients—either directly or indirectly—and I do it only when there is an immediate need to rapidly interrupt and disrupt the entrenched trance response pattern.

Perhaps the easiest way to get a sense of oppositional trances is to work with couples. One typical presentation comes in the form of the wife complaining that her husband is never around; he's always at work, and even when he is at home, he isn't available on any level. The husband claims to be under a lot of pressure at work, and believes he has no other choice but to act in this way.

In reality, you are witnessing the dynamic interaction of two oppositional trances: the wife is in a chronic trance state of over-identification, while the husband is hidden away in a comfortable cloak of dissociation. Many forms of therapy work with this prototypical couples' problem by layering various posthypnotic suggestions over the trance states: the husband will be encouraged to learn how to become more emotionally present, and the wife will be encouraged to cultivate outside interests of her own. Encouragement will come in the form of verbal discussion and therapeutic injunctions. The problem with such an approach is that the words often cannot penetrate the entrenched trance state. The trance itself must be shifted or altered before the words will have a "receptacle."

Case Example

Janice and Joe began their first couples' session with the complaint we are discussing: "Joe is never home; Joe is never available"...."Janice is too clingy; Janice is too dependent on me." The husband was noticeably dissociated, as he sat in a sprawling "I-couldn't-care-less" posture on the couch and made it clear that he was only there "to get some peace and quiet." The wife, meanwhile, was leaning toward her sprawled out husband, trying with every word she spoke to engage his interest.

It was obvious to me that it would be futile to try to work with the husband's trance directly. He didn't want to be *here*, period. So I turned my focus to the wife and began to work with her trance of over-identification. My eventual goal was that she learn to dissociate somewhat from her husband, but I did not want to give her direct suggestions for dissociation. Instead, I began by indirectly suggesting another trance state, that of hypnotic dreaming, by asking her simply, "What are your dreams? If you could do *anything*, what are your dreams?"

She answered that she had always wanted to have her own small business. She wanted to take courses and learn how to do it.

I spent the rest of the session facilitating and supporting Janice's trance of hypnotic dreaming, helping her to vivify her dream. I didn't address the husband at any point. To close, I gave Janice the homework assignment of calling at least one place every day for a job, and investigating training schools.

By the next session, the husband presented an entirely different impression. He sat composed and alert and began discussing his discomfort with his wife's new behavior. Clearly, he was no longer in his chronic trance state of dissociation. By facilitating Janice's shift out of her over-identified trance into a new trance that produced opposing behavior, Joe's own chronic trance of dissociation was shifted—without once being directly addressed.

Case Example

A man in his forties, a former business executive, came to therapy with a presenting problem of exhibitionism—he was a flasher. He had been through the court system, he had been to seven different therapists, but nothing seemed to work. His appraisal was "I'm over 40—I'm too old to change."

During the first session he gave me all the appropriate etiological history: how as a little boy, he would show his penis to his mommy, and she thought it was cute and funny. So, he was still doing it—still trying to recreate mommy's delight in him. By the end of the session I had a strong intuitive sense that it was futile to try to work with this man one-on-one. I asked him to bring his wife to the next session. He agreed.

I began by interviewing him for a quick five minutes, and then turned my attention to the wife—who was more than willing to communicate. She stated that, although in her forties, she had never had an orgasm because her husband was the "wham-bam-thank-you-ma'am" type. I perceived their oppositional trances to be dissociation (the wife) and over-identification (the husband). The husband's trance of over-identification became sublimated into flashing because his wife no longer wanted to have sex with him.

I discontinued therapy with the man while I worked exclusively with the wife. I focused on shifting her trance of dissociation to one of over-identification, while increasing her experience of sensation. She was not willing to masturbate and could not even tolerate the word, so I called it "making love with yourself"—which she was very interested in doing.

After four weeks of sessions, continually increasing the flow of sensations (as well as referring her for Feldenkrais sessions), she became orgasmic; meanwhile, her husband's exhibitionism was *decreasing*. As amazing as it sounds, the more sexual she became, the less need he felt to expose himself or sublimate his over-identification. At that point I asked him to come back into the sessions and "help" (this word was used to preserve his much needed one-up status) his wife explore her new world. In addition I worked with him for several sessions, primarily asking him to exaggerate his flashing by using his whole body in my office. Eventually, the flashing disappeared altogether. I believe it was this systems approach to hypnotherapy—the recognition that the symptom was context-dependent—that created the transforming shift.

Case Example

I recently worked with a woman whose father had repeatedly locked her in a dry well when she was a little girl. As a result, her body was still feeling pain in 1986. I understood that the experiencing of pain from 25 years ago was partly due to the Deep Trance Phenomenon of over-identification, whereby she remained attached to the trauma in a "frozen" and age-regressed manner. Her legs still felt paralyzed and painful at the same time. Consequently, I taught her dissociation. In a sense, development of the oppositional trance adds water to the glue of current Deep Trance Phenomena that are holding the symptom structure together.

Table 2
Oppositional Trances

Age Regression .... Pseudo-Orientation in Time
Amnesia .... Hypermnesia
Analgesia .... Sensory Distortion
Dissociation .... Over-Identification
Hypnotic Dreaming .... Over-Identification
Negative Hallucination .... Positive Hallucination

Treatment of Dissociation

The treatment of dissociation is probably the most direct of all the Deep Trance Phenomena:

Step 1: If the client brings you dissociation as the symptomatic trance, ask him to continue to dissociate *as he breathes and looks at you*. This allows the client to experience his symptom in an interpersonal context, which automatically expands the focus.

Step 2: Ask the client to "start and stop" the dissociation by allowing himself to "space out" for a few minutes, followed by a few minutes of intense conversation with you. Continue to alternate in this fashion: spacing out, followed by focused interaction. This alternation gives the client his first experience of having conscious control over the automatic response of dissociation.

> *Axiom: If you consciously and intentionally create a trance in present time, you take charge of it and strip it of its autonomous, symptomatic quality.*

10

Posthypnotic Suggestion

POSTHYPNOTIC SUGGESTIONS are the cornerstone of reality formation. How we experience the outer world of people and events as well as the internal world of affective states is largely shaped by this powerful Deep Trance Phenomenon. The child adapts to early threat by internalizing the parents' posthypnotic suggestions. These are then put on automatic, which means that the child, adolescent, teenager, young adult, continues to self-suggest limiting behavioral inevitabilities out of context. Eventually, these posthypnotic suggestions coalesce into some kind of symptom structure. Unless the individual gains the power of choice over the internal auditory dialogues (posthypnotic suggestions) that rule her in the present, she will never experience freedom from entrenched family ideology and pathology.

As with all Deep Trance Phenomena, posthypnotic suggestion is created by a series of *inter*personal interactions (parent-to-child) that are eventually internalized as *intra*personal communications (self-to-self) in the form of introjects or what we might call "auditory dialogues." In essence, parents communicate messages to children, either verbally or nonverbally, which children internalize and put on automatic. Some of these messages may be helpful to the child's developing self-image; many are detrimental. Most endure well into adulthood and are inevitably part of whatever symptomatology emerges.

Most people imagine posthypnotic suggestion to be quite magical, as when the stage hypnotist instructs the volunteer, "When I snap my fingers, you will be a chicken." This is a primitive form of posthypnotic suggestion; parents are far more sophisticated in their application of this Deep Trance Phenomenon. Parental post-hypnotic suggestions such as "Men will hurt you" or "You'll never get what you want" are shaped into core beliefs by the child that then proceed to influence an entire lifetime.

In traditional hypnotic work posthypnotic suggestion is used to assess the effectiveness of trance and reinforce the therapeutic change that has occurred during the session (Erickson & Rossi, 1979). Typically, a patient is given a suggestion to behave in a certain way after she is out of the trance and back in real life. Her behavioral compliance supposedly ratifies the therapeutic trance—and proves what a good hypnotist the practitioner is.

As hypnotherapy evolved through Erickson's contributions, the definition, content, and form of posthypnotic suggestions also evolved (Erickson & Rossi, 1979):

> In the broadest sense we can speak of posthypnotic sugges-tion whenever we introduce an idea during a moment of receptivity that is later actualized in behavior. That moment of receptivity can occur during a formally induced trance or during the *common everyday trance* in which attention is fixed and absorbed in a matter of great interest. (p. 85)

Erickson and Rossi (1979) explain the difference between tradi-tional posthypnotic suggestion and Ericksonian methods:

> The traditional approach to direct posthypnotic suggestion usually takes the form, "After you awaken from trance, you will do [or experience] such and such." Indirect posthyp-notic suggestion, by contrast, [utilizes] inevitable patterns of behavior that the patient will experience in the future. . . .The patient's own associations, life experience, personality dynamics, and future prospects are all utilized to build the posthypnotic suggestion into the patient's natural life structure. (pp. 85-86)

Using Erickson's expanded view of posthypnotic suggestion as "an idea [offered] during a moment of receptivity that is later actualized in behavior" makes it easy to see the degree to which our childhoods are quite literally strewn with the carcasses of this Deep Trance Phenomenon.

Erickson's *Collected Papers*, together with all the Erickson/ Rossi volumes, can be studied for numerous, rich examples of his permissive-utilization approach to posthypnotic suggestion.

My approach to posthypnotic suggestion offers another alternative. Not surprisingly, it follows the principle of *utilizing the Deep Trance Phenomena* presented by patients as part of their symptomatology. In this case, I am going to utilize their own verbatim posthypnotic suggestions to create new suggestions.

What kinds of posthypnotic suggestions do clients bring us? Thousands of them! Most of us have had a good 15-20 years of exposure to two very powerful hypnotists: our parents. Although the giving of posthypnotic suggestion is an inextricable part of parenting, most parents do not realize their powerful roles as hypnotists. Also problematic are the conflicting hypnotic messages mothers and fathers often unknowingly present: the mother's trance induction and posthypnotic suggestions are opposite those the father gives. Talk about naturalistic confusion trances!

For example, the mother might tell her little girl, in essence, "You're pretty, you have pretty eyes and pretty hair, and you're so sweet. . . .You'll probably always get what you want. . . .You can have anything you want. . . .You will do very well in school, and I really like the way you can read. . . .You're really studying hard, and you can have whatever you want."

These suggestions are given on a daily basis in one form or another and constitute one body of posthypnotic suggestions to which the child is exposed.

Meanwhile, Dad comes along with his overriding message (trance induction) of, in essence, *Women are dumb and your place is in the home.* His little girl (adolescent, teenager) regularly and repetitiously hears things like: "Women don't really make it in the world. . . .They're not very bright. . . .You've got blonde hair, and you know what men think of girls with blonde hair. . . .My mother stayed home to raise her kids, and your mother stays at home to raise you, and I think it's a damn good idea for women to be in the home. . . . You're safe here, in this home, and I'm a good provider. You don't need anything more than that. It's so nice that your mother doesn't have to work and that I can look after her. . . . She doesn't have to have a career and you don't have to have a career when you grow up. I know you want to go to college, and you might just do that some day, but it would be better to meet a doctor or lawyer and get married."

The child is thus confronted with two conflicting sets of posthypnotic suggestions that give rise to intrapersonal conflict and conflicted behavioral responses. Further complicating this dynamic is the fact that the suggestions are linked to things she sees everyday, and many are even part of her physical make-up (Erickson and Rossi's "behavioral inevitabilities" [Erickson & Rossi, 1979; Erickson, Rossi, & Rossi, 1987]): eyes, hair, face, books, home. With repetition and consistency, the posthypnotic trance messages of both parents are internalized and put on automatic, dominating the child's inner experience through adolescence, teen years, and well in to adulthood.

I have talked about how the child internalizes many of the posthypnotic suggestions proffered by the parents. This process of internalization can be further broken down into three separate categories:

(1) the child *goes into agreement* with the suggestions;
(2) the child *resists* the suggestions;
(3) or, the child *duplicates* the suggestions.

A young girl who gets a message from her father that she is unattractive—which she experiences on an unconscious level as a posthypnotic suggestion of "I'm ugly"—might *go into agreement* with the suggestion and become an overweight child and an acne-ridden teenager. Here, she immerses herself in the experience of "I'm ugly," as well as the concomitant judgment of "It's bad to be ugly." It is the ongoing presence of this judgment, "It's bad to be ugly," that causes the person's distress and symptomatic problems.

Another response possibility is to *resist* the suggestion and create a counter one of "I'm beautiful." Like the above child, this child judges the experience of "I'm ugly" to be bad, but unlike the other child, she is unwilling to experience it. So she creates its opposite. But the voice that says "No, I'm not ugly" is continually responding to the voice that says, "I'm ugly and that's bad." So it is a perpetual double bind. No matter how hard the child/woman works at being beautiful, and no matter how close she comes to being beautiful, the underlying suggestion, "I'm ugly," remains in her consciousness.

The third possible response of *duplication* is really an ideal— I think it would only be possible for a "zen child"—a child reared in a carefully controlled environment that taught him/her from Day One *not* to judge, only to *be*. In this response modality, a child told that he is ugly places no negative judgment on being ugly and so is completely willing to experience the experience labeled "I'm ugly." No later problems crop up, because there was no negative judgment on the experience and hence no resistance of it. I know, I know, only in the television reruns of *Kung Fu*, where Grasshopper learns to walk on rice paper and leave no tracks. I mention duplication, however, because it *is* a potential way of responding—perhaps one that we are just beginning to learn how to cultivate.

Principles (Axioms) of Posthypnotic Suggestion

A developing child is deluged with hundreds of posthypnotic suggestions, delivered by well-meaning as well as abusive parents. Not *all* of these are internalized. Now we are going to examine two factors, or axioms, that help determine whether or not a posthypnotic suggestion is internalized. Both axioms contain elements from the field of learning theory that are then placed in a new context of hypnotic learning. Here behavior is not viewed as a straightforward product of the stimulus-response equation, but as a complex circuitry involving stimulus-response mechanisms in dynamic interaction with Deep Trance Phenomena as they manifest out of each person's unique life experience.

Axiom I: An experience once resisted persists until the person is willing to "experience the experience."

The phenomenon of resistance is the foundation of most psycho-emotional symptomatology. Resistance to painful experience paradoxically fuels and sustains the very experience we try so hard to avoid, ignore, wish away. In essence, all the "voices" that badger us within our own minds are resisted experiences. Posthypnotic suggestions gain their foothold through the soil of resistance, which provides ample nutrients for their growth.

Let's use a simple example to break down the process by which posthypnotic suggestions are implanted.

Dad comes upon his four-year-old son, who is busily trying to turn on the complicated television set in the large, looming wood cabinet. Disgruntled, the father snaps, "How many times do I have to tell you not to touch that! You don't know how to operate it. Now stay away!"

Four-year-olds do not stay away, however, nor do five-, six-, or seven-year-olds. The scene is repeated dozens of times in this young child's life, and each time the child resists (tenses against) experiencing the father's negative communications that tell the child he "doesn't know how" and "stay away." On an unconscious level, the child incorporates both of these messages (posthypnotic suggestions) into his personal world view about himself. The *I don't know* and *stay away* injunctions may then generalize to all other mechanical/electrical devices—VCRs, computers, radios, lawnmowers, even cars.

Ideally, the young child receiving reprimands learns and lets go of them. In reality, however, most parenting is too rushed to provide the kind of message-giving that would make it possible for a child to run through a complete learning circuit without forming a negative belief about herself, embedded as a posthypnotic suggestion. Statements are tossed out, injunctions are given; the young child bristles against them—resists them—thus paradoxically preserving their presence and influence in his life. Our hypothetical child, above, soon internalizes the parent's message (posthypnotic suggestion) and is therefore constantly working *against* it. Each situation involving the right trigger stimulus (a mechanical/electrical device) will evoke the original posthypnotic suggestions—*you don't understand* and *stay away* —and their accompanying resistance.

Another brief example, easy for many of us to relate to, is the parental injunction, "Work hard." Almost every child is taught that working hard is a virtue, but not every child complies with the teaching. A resistant child, who experiences his parents as uncaring and inattentive, might create the response "That's bullshit" to the posthypnotic suggestion, "Work hard." The child then spends the rest of his life proving his father wrong by himself creating an opposing lifestyle. This involves two simultaneous trances: his internalized parental identity trance ("Work hard"), and a counter-identity trance ("Bullshit"). Constant internal conflict is the net result.

> *Axiom II: An experience that occurs consistently following a pleasant outcome will become part of the person's belief system in a literal and repetitive manner.*

This axiom nicely complements the first; it is yet another common way in which posthypnotic suggestions get internalized. As an example, let's say a young child is sitting at the kitchen table, agonizing over learning his letters. At the end of his homework session, Dad pats him on the back and says, "See, if you work hard, you can do anything."

The pleasant outcome is the child's completion of his homework assignment coupled with his father's approval. This is then paired with the injunction to work hard. When such an experience is consistently presented to a child—when approval is repeatedly wedded to an injunction—he or she will begin to seek approval obsessively. The posthypnotic suggestion, "Work hard," once triggered in relation to learning the letters of the alphabet, is now triggered with a vast array of stimuli—salary, money in general, the boss's approval, the spouse's approval, job evaluations, and so on. The resulting experience is one of feeling driven and, at the same, that nothing he does is ever quite enough.

It is important to understand that while posthypnotic suggestions have a verbal content—we think of them in terms of *words*—they are first and foremost a communication, a message, a view of reality, that can be communicated on entirely nonverbal levels. For example, a quiet, reclusive parent who almost never inquires about the child's well-being might be communicating the posthypnotic suggestion, "Nobody is interested in you." That is to say, "nobody is interested in you" is how the child interprets the behavior. The child infers through the nonverbal cuing of silence a particular message and then creates an intrapersonal trance that is in accord with her interpretation of the interpersonal context.

Fusion, Yea or Nea

In Chapter 1 we touched on the topic of trance identities that will be elaborated in Chapters 14 and 19. These identities are trance states created when the child, for purposes of survival, fuses with a particular experience. In this chapter we can begin to talk in more detail about the means by which these trance identities are formed: the internalization of posthypnotic suggestion, on both verbal and nonverbal levels. This internalization creates a trance state of fusion between parent and child that narrows and rigidifies the child's developing sense of self.

The impetus for fusion can flow in two directions: from parent to child, or from child to parent. In the first case, the parent pressures the child to "be just like me," or some variation thereof. In the second, the child will create the fusion as a fantasized solution to a threatening environment: "If I'm just like Mom, everything will work out okay." This dynamic is particularly fascinating in cases of abuse: the child will actually fuse with the abusive parent in an attempt to handle the attack. As mentioned previously, this same dynamic underlies the incest survivor's fusion with the perpetrator. This is kind of a psychological Aikido. One becomes the perpetrator to resist the onslaughts.

Let's break the process down, step by step.

Dad, for one reason or another, consistently communicates the message, "Be just like me," to his young son. The child incorporates the message and then responds to it with either compliance or resistance. If he complies with it, the child, in effect, ends up *resisting his own personality* which is not allowed, and acting out his father's personality. If he resists the injunction, "Be just like me," he ends up with a resisting identity that is in continual conflict with the father's personality. Even if the child resists Dad and creates a "new life," he must always carry "Dad" in his psyche so that he knows what to resist. The internalized father is then projected, possibly onto authority figures, whom he feels he must always resist.

Let's back up. In both cases of compliance and resistance, *two* conflicting trance identities are formed in childhood: a fused-father identity, and a resisted-father identity. Also in both cases, these trance identities will persist into adulthood and be projected upon an ever continuing array of appropriate figures.

The child who resists Dad's pressure will form, over time, a resisting identity; this identity may come in the form of a negative rebuff ("Fuck you, Dad") or a positive assertion ("I'm going to be myself"). This resisting identity sits side-by-side with the fused identity it is opposing ("I'm just like Dad").

However hard the child/adult tries to "just be myself," the fused identity will remain in robust—if grossly projected—form. Typically, the adult who has resisted his father's injunction to "be just like me" will project this demand (the fused identity) on all authority figures. Every teacher, every boss, perhaps even most older men, will be resisted, fought, and pushed away to one degree or another. No matter how the person actually behaves, he will be labeled and therefore experienced as a fused-father identity. In essence, the adult goes about creating identities for all these people, regardless of their real identities—*just like his father did when he disallowed the child's personality in favor of superimposing his own.* Now the adult is superimposing a personality—his internalized fused trance identity with his father—and seeing all these other people as trying to force him to be like them.

The child who goes into compliance with the fused identity goes through a similar process with slightly different content. This child has denied his own self or ego and he now experiences life through the eyes, ears, thoughts, and perceptual experiences of the father. This child will grow into an adult who never knows why he is frustrated or discontented, since he always does the "right thing—just like Dad." This brings us to our next axiom.

Axiom III: When a fused identity is resisted, a resisting identity is formed.

Choice Point: The New Horizon

Throughout this book I have said that each Deep Trance Phenomenon is selected and created by a child as a means of ensuring his/her survival. I would like to emphasize that this does not mean that the child is a victim, haplessly attaching himself to this Deep Trance Phenomenon or that. . .internalizing this set of posthypnotic suggestions or that set. I do not ascribe to the traditional scenario in which Mom and Dad are scapegoated as the "blame-ees" and the abused child is seen as the victimized "blame-er."

In my view, an important level of choice always exists. On one level, the child at the level of being chooses whether she goes into agreement with the posthypnotic suggestions presented by her parents, whether she resists, or whether she duplicates. She chooses her response at all times, and in all ways. It's not what Mommy and Daddy have done to us that continues to haunt us; it is what we as free beings *create* in response to them. This concept is elaborated in great detail in my forthcoming book, *Quantum Consciousness: The Discovery and Birth of Quantum Psychology: The Physics of Consciousness*. Briefly stated, the observer (you) creates the experience of that which is observed. This interpretation of physicist Werner Heisenberg's "Uncertainty Principle," which is the cutting-edge in the creation of Quantum Psychology, is discussed further by Nick Herbert in his book, *Quantum Reality,* in which Herbert discusses the Copenhagen Interpretation Part II (reality is created by observation). For now, suffice it to say that *our experience of reality is observer created*. Why? Because at the level of being, each of us chooses to create a response to posthypnotic suggestions and behaviors. This profound understanding empowers the individual and engenders a deeper level of responsibility than just handling psychological material.

If my father repeatedly communicates to me, verbally and nonverbally, "You are inadequate," that is *his* creation, *his* posthypnotic suggestion, *his* "thought-form," if you will. Even as a child, I possess an inner autonomy of response, and that response constitutes my own self-created posthypnotic suggestion. What we need to understand is that *this process is a creative one*: In response to my father I either go into agreement with him, or I oppose him. If I go into agreement, it means that *I create* a corroborating posthypnotic suggestion or series of suggestions. At this point I also create a corresponding mental picture of how I think Dad sees me, and then I place it on "auto pilot" to sustain this image with which I have gone into collusion. Or, I resist his suggestion and create an opposing one: "I don't want to be like him, no matter what!" At that point I, as a being, take a picture of Dad and place it on "auto pilot" in my consciousness so that I continuously remind myself of what I am *not* to become.

Either way, *choice* and *creativity* are involved.

I am aware that this view seems to oversimplify things. You are probably protesting, "But a *child* isn't really free...A child is totally vulnerable, totally dependent, and so that makes parents responsible." But what if, in the larger picture, on some level of awareness we but dimly glimpse, each child is precisely free to choose its reactions to the environment in which it lives? I include these thoughts only to emphasize how we hold beliefs we assume are "reality," when in fact they are based only on a set of assumptions no more provable than other assumptions. There is a point at which therapists must consciously face the issue of the degree to which they believe in the concept of *victim*. We are all confronted by it; I am simply sharing my own personal response to that exploration.

Clients thus arrive for therapy carrying varying amounts of posthypnotic baggage, manifesting in the form of a particular symptom or problem. A therapist who employs therapeutic hypnosis will typically use trance to give suggestions that offer solutions, alternatives, the evocation of inner resources, and so on. An Ericksonian hypnotherapy session is typically characterized by a permissive and naturalistic style (rather than authoritarian) that gives the client a series of posthypnotic suggestions utilizing "the patient's own associations, life experience, personality dynamics, and future prospects. . . ."

My use of posthypnotic suggestion differs markedly from both classical and Ericksonian methods. I take the parental posthypnotic suggestions the client has verbalized during our discussions, either knowingly or unknowingly, and utilize those very suggestions to shift the trance state.

Case Example

A young woman whose main issue was an inability to be intimate described her parents as being extremely unaffectionate with one another as well as with their children. In her descriptions they sounded almost phobic about physical demonstrations of love of any kind. The posthypnotic suggestions inherent in the client's parents' behavior ran something like: "Don't touch me....Don't be close. . . .Don't love me. . . .Don't care about me." I took these suggestions and split them into two different hypnotic voices that opened up completely new alternatives without superimposing anything. *By using shifts in eye contact and vocal tone together with pauses, the original posthypnotic suggestions can be bifurcated into two separate realities: one embodies the old reality of **don'ts**, while the other points to a new reality of **do**.*

I began by vocalizing the posthypnotic suggestions with their original meaning intact: "Don't touch me, don't love me, don't come near me, don't care about me." Then I shifted the entire experience, retaining the words verbatim, but subtly altering all covert levels of communication.

Looking into her left eye I said softly, almost inaudibly, "*Don't.*" Now shifting to look directly into her right eye, I said more emphatically, "**Be close to me.**" I repeated the suggestion and included all related versions:

Don't	**Be close to me**
Don't	**Touch me**
Don't	**Come near me**

With this use of carefully modulated vocal cues and eye contact, I have shifted the trance by shifting the emphasis on the posthypnotic suggestions. I have also shifted the trance by *taking over* the posthypnotic suggestions: I'm saying all those things, so she doesn't have to do them to herself; I am doing them for her—which leaves her extremely receptive to a new message, which is really an old message: her desire for intimacy. I'm teasing out her wish, her need for intimacy, which is a resource she was not allowed to develop. *The therapist thus becomes the container for the old posthypnotic suggestions and, at the same time, the catalyst for the new.*

Treatment of Posthypnotic Suggestion

I. *Recording.* Begin unraveling your own posthypnotic trance states by simply writing down or tape-recording the posthypnotic suggestions you give to yourself. Obviously, you can't go through your whole day scribbling away on a note pad, so for focus, pick any problem area in your life. Say you tend to get extremely anxious over money issues, or whenever you have to meet with your boss, or each time you wake up in the middle of the night. Take this circumscribed opportunity to study *how you are putting yourself into the trance of fear and anxiety.*

Another way to "tease out" your posthypnotic suggestions is to state out loud the opposite of what you are feeling: For example, if you are worried about money you might state, "I have plenty of money," or "I am financially secure," and then notice what posthypnotic suggestions pop up for you. You might have a counter response of, "But I *don't* have plenty of money—I'm *in debt and I'll never* get out of it." Or you might find yourself scoffing that "There's no such thing as financial security."

This simple act of writing down your own posthypnotic suggestions is surprisingly powerful because it immediately distances you from those suggestions. Typically, you are completely identified with the state called "I hate myself," or "I'm terrified"; you stand in the middle of the suggestion or thought-form, surrounded by it, believing it is the total picture of reality. Once you place yourself in the observer mode of the witnessing relationship, however, *you* expand. Instead of *being* the suggestion, you are now *watching* your suggestion. This means that your relationship to the suggestion has already changed drastically. *The perceiver is not the perceived. If you can perceive your posthypnotic suggestions, then obviously you are not them; your reality extends beyond them.*

Let's say that you awaken one morning feeling "blah." That's as descriptive as you can be about your state. You just feel blah, and you don't like it. One way to work with it is simply to be with it for a few minutes. Lie down in a comfortable position and focus on the sensations that comprise the blah feeling by re-creating in your mind's eye your very first moments upon awakening. Notice what you say to yourself and write down what comes up, for example:

"Life's hard. It's Sunday and I've got nothing to do. I'm so bored, what am I going to do all day? I feel empty. . . .My life is empty. Most people look forward to the weekend; there must be something wrong with me."

Voila, *blah!*

Gradually, if you practice this exercise consistently, you will begin to become fascinated by your own autohypnotic abilities. We all hypnotize ourselves on a daily basis, yet most of us firmly believe we know nothing about self-hypnosis. We know everything about it—all we have to do is watch, look, listen—to *ourselves.*

Now that you have placed yourself outside of the suggestion, note that you are disidentified from it and therefore can begin to work with it.

II. *Splitting*. My approach to working with posthypnotic suggestions is entirely *process oriented*. As I mentioned in a previous chapter, I am not interested in the working with the content or storyline that is viewed as being the causal agent of the posthypnotic suggestion. For me, the causal agent can be found in the present moment, in the self-to-self trance the individual is actively creating and sustaining.

The technique of splitting is an excellent example of the difference between content- and process-oriented approaches. As the case example above illustrated, the goal is to split apart the suggestions in order to emphasize the resource inherent in them. So, as we saw, the posthypnotic suggestion of "Don't trust people" is not discussed from the historical, experiential point of view—it is simply worked with as a force in present time. When a therapist is using this technique, eye contact and shifts in voice are used to emphasize the splitting now being imposed between the negative injunction of DON'T, and the positive injunction of TRUST PEOPLE.

To use the technique of splitting by yourself, begin by lying down and getting comfortable and quiet. Focus all your attention on the inner sensation of the suggestion, DON'T TRUST PEOPLE. Feel it; notice what subtle changes happen in your body. Now begin splitting the word DON'T from the words TRUST PEOPLE. Change the inflection in your inner voice so that DON'T begins to sound softer, while TRUST PEOPLE is said with strength and good feeling. Allow yourself to revel in the inner sensation of the words TRUST PEOPLE, noting as you do so all the pleasant, subtle changes throughout your body. You are beginning to experience this long-buried resource called TRUST PEOPLE in your physical body; you have removed all the weeds and seeded it within yourself.

By taking the original experience created by the posthypnotic suggestion called "Don't trust people" and changing it via inflection and emphasis, you create its opposite experience, which is a welcome resource.

III. *Questions.* Take your list of self-delivered posthypnotic suggestions and *turn them into questions.*

I hate my myself?
I don't want to live?
Nothing works?
I'm a worthless loser?

By turning the statements into questions, a number of changes occur. First, you create a kind of doubt (a question automatically implies the existence of doubt); second, in order to change the statement into a question, you have to create a kind of secondary level of awareness which separates the perceiver from the perceived; and third, it stimulates you to retrieve resources that were not available a moment or two ago.

IV. *Creating Multiple Meanings.* This technique is probably easier to do with a therapist, but it can also be highly effective for an individual working alone. Basically, you take what I call trigger words—*hate, don't trust, don't touch*—that are the core of your posthypnotic suggestions and you create multiple meanings and completely new associations. With each new suggestion, allow yourself to drift into a sleepy state where resources and symbols can begin to emerge. For example, the posthypnotic suggestion

I hate myself

is reassociated with several new meanings

I rate myself
I create myself
I date myself.

At first glance this may sound like semantic mumbo-jumbo, but it actually can bring about significant alterations in one's perception of the original posthypnotic suggestion by creating confusion which absorbs the focus of attention of the conscious mind—thus allowing unconscious resources to emerge. In essence, you are creating additional meanings and ideas *which dilute and disperse the single-pointed focus of the original meaning* ("I hate myself"). You are also creating a subtle trance of confusion which, in effect, depotentiates your conscious rational thinking and allows the nonrational processes of your unconscious mind to flow—whereupon resources and symbols begin to emerge spontaneously and completely naturalistically.

In conclusion, posthypnotic suggestions are the words that are used to create an internal symptom. In classical hypnosis words such as *relax, comfort, sleep, tired* are superimposed over the client's symptom state in an effort to bring about the outcome of relaxation. In my approach symptomatic posthypnotic suggestions are the source of symptomatic outcomes and therefore become the pivotal point of intervention.

11

Amnesia

AMNESIA has received a lot of press lately, only under a different name: *denial*. Co-dependent groups everywhere speak about abuse and denial as opposite sides of the same coin of addiction. *Denial* as a primary experience within the family is on everyone's lips.

Long before the widespread awareness of denial, there was amnesia. Amnesia has been around a very long time, and holds an honored place in the history of hypnosis. To understand just how honored—and central—a position it holds, let's take a brief look at the history of amnesia.

James Braid (1795-1860), one of the earliest investigators of hypnosis, actually defined hypnosis in terms of the amnesia that so typically surrounded it (Rossi, 1986): "Let the term *hypnotism* be restricted to those cases alone in which. . .the subject has no remembrance on awakening of what occurred during his sleep, but of which he shall have the most perfect recollection on passing into a similar stage of hypnotism thereafter" (p. 36). Braid's successor, Pierre Janet, considered amnesia and its attendant dissociation to be the very source of psychopathology. This paved the way for the embryonic psychoanalytic view posited by Freud, who saw repressed memories as the basis of psychogenic problems. Jung, meanwhile, investigated "complexes" through his word association tests, concluding that "forgetting normally takes place at or immediately after disturbance caused by a complex." Indeed, according to Rossi (1986), "the entire edifice of psychoanalysis could be said to rest upon this effort to explain how trauma gave rise to emotional complexes by initiating dissociation, repressions, and amnesias" (p. 39).

Rossi (1986) goes on to summarize his and Erickson's overview of the history and nature of therapeutic hypnosis: "Taken together, these clinical and naturalistic investigations strongly suggest that hypnotic trance is an altered *state* of consciousness, and amnesia, in particular, is a natural consequence of this altered state" (p. 40).

Thus, in the course of amnesia's illustrious career, it has been viewed as the core of traditional hypnosis, the core of psychopathology in general, the core of Freudian psychoanalysis, the core of Jungian complexes, and the core of modern-day Ericksonian hypnosis. Amnesia is like a revolving doorway: ever spinning, but pushed one way by one person, and another way by another person. Sometimes it is responsible for the bad effects of repression; sometimes it is applauded for its positive effects in hypnosis. One could get vertigo, investigating this puzzle called amnesia.

Erickson first made us aware of the "common everyday" experiences of amnesia we all accrue on a regular basis: Forgetting the time of your dentist appointment, forgetting the date of your mother-in-law's birthday, forgetting the time of a dreaded cocktail party, and so forth. *Forgetting* is probably one of the most common experiences we share as humans. However, when we experience it as a regular—and problematic—part of our lives, it is probably because the process of forgetting has been upgraded to the an autonomous trance state of amnesia.

How does normal forgetting grow into a symptomatic trance state? In the same fashion as other Deep Trance Phenomena are birthed: as a means of preserving, protecting, or supporting the child in the context of early family experiences that cannot be processed. Chronic amnesic states—which include the complimentary trance state of hypermnesia—are intense efforts to maintain the homeostasis of the individual and/or the environment. In my view of amnesia, it is not so much a consequence of the altered state of hypnosis as it is *itself* a full-fledged trance state; the sensation of being in hypnosis arises *out of* ongoing amnesic trance states, not the other way around.

This brings us back to the point of utilizing the particular trance state that the patient brings to the session versus inducing another trance state deemed to be therapeutic. Erickson typically induced amnesia for trance work in the hope of protecting any therapeutic effects from the barrage of conscious, critical thought processes. In my approach, the critical thought processes are themselves the product of dynamic, interactive trance phenomena which are at the root of the symptom. Therefore, rather than trying to bypass them, I would invite the Deep Trance Phenomena out into the open, so to speak.

Let me add that inducing amnesia may be indicated on occasion, but it is definitely not necessary in the majority of cases. In working with an alcoholic woman, I suggested that she have amnesia for all our trance work. She experienced so much amnesia that after two-and-a-half months of not drinking, she reported that there were "no changes" in her life and wondered if she was making progress. On an unconscious level she knew the answer, but on a conscious level, the amnesia functioned as a means of continually distancing alcoholism as a problem in her life.

Naturalistic suggestions for the experience of amnesia may also be given to a person who is severely hypermnesic, as a means of accelerating a balance between the two states. An example of this type of suggestion might be:

> "How pleasant it is to remember unpleasant situations, realizing how much you have learned. And your conscious mind can eat the 'food,' and your unconscious mind can digest it. Your unconscious mind already knows what it needs to keep the body fit and healthy, and it knows what to eliminate; what you don't really need anymore."

Another naturalistic suggestion for amnesia, often used to counterbalance entrenched hypermnesia, might be:

> "I feel like a breeze flowing through the woods. As the breeze goes through the woods, ideas can flow in one ear and out the other ear, and where did the breeze go, and

where did the leaves go? Did they disappear into the breeze?"

Amnesia is a survival mechanism, a naturalistic mode of defense birthed in early childhood. We tend to think about amnesia as a *cognitive* state when, in fact, it is very much a *body* state. When an adult arrives for therapy with the complaint, "I just can't remember my childhood," she will also exhibit physical cues such as shallow breathing and rigid musculature. Watch for these, and then ask the client to breathe and look at you as she re-creates her trance state of amnesia. Following is a partial transcript of a demonstration before a group of student-professionals.

> *Therapist*: I want you to remember a time when you felt amnesic. Can you see an image of yourself over here, in that situation?
> *Client*: [Spoken softly, as if in slow-motion] I see "Bull-dog."
> *Therapist*: Who is Bull-Dog?
> *Client*: The class bully—that was his nickname.
> *Therapist*: The class bully. Okay. I'd like you to continue to look at Bull-Dog as you breathe and look at me. . .as you breathe and look at me. I'd like you to see Bull-Dog, describe him as minutely as possible, and bring him back with you into the present.
> *Client*: [Squirms in chair, breathing becomes erratic, forehead is deeply furrowed.]
> *Therapist*: What is happening in your body when you re-create Bull-Dog in present time?
> *Client*: I remember being beaten up.

Another client complained of being forgetful throughout the day, in a very generalized but disturbing way.

> *Therapist*: Tell me what happens if you imagine yourself unable to remember something in a present-day situation.
> *Client*: Yes, I can see it.
> *Therapist*: If you were to pull the image of yourself *remembering* back inside of you, what would happen?
> *Client*: I feel stupid.

Therapist: You feel stupid. And what is happening in your body, in your muscles?
Client: I'm giving it all, holding back right here [gestures slowly to stomach area].
Therapist: [To audience] She has given you a clue for a wonderful posthypnotic suggestion about feeling stupid. [To client] Did you hear what you said?
Client: I didn't hear what I said.
Therapist: Living proof of amnesia! So as you continue to breathe and look at me, you might. . .notice the tightness of the stomach, the voice inside that says "I'm stupid. . .I can't. . .remember. . .I can't. . .remember anything."

In order to experience amnesia, the client in our above example has to stop breathing, tighten her stomach and say to herself, "I'm stupid...I can't remember." By first appreciating her amnesia and then working with the body trance and splitting the posthypnotic suggestions (*see Chapter 10*), you interrupt the normal pathway that culminates in her amnesia.

Another fascinating concept, which cradles amnesia at its core, is the concept of hypnosis as a state-dependent phenomenon. According to Rossi (1986), Braid's quotation implies the concept of state-dependent phenomena without naming it as such. When an experience is "state-dependent," it means that it will be remembered only with the return of the altered state of consciousness that accompanied it. Thus, a person involved in a serious auto accident will tend to have great difficulty recalling the sequence of traumatic events once he or she has re-entered "normal" consciousness. Recall will become more accessible, however, whenever arousal physiology is triggered in the person's body.

Researchers have been talking about the state-dependent quality of drug experiences for a couple of decades now. Only recently has Rossi (1986; Rossi & Cheek, 1988), picking up the thread of Braid's early implication, elaborated a theory of hypnosis as a state-dependent behavior.

In previous chapters I have consistently described Deep Trance Phenomena as "context-independent"—which *sounds* like the opposite of "state-dependent," but isn't. All symptomatic Deep Trance

Phenomena are state-dependent *as well as* context-independent. Because Deep Trance Phenomena are *physical* experiences, they are accompanied by specific physiological characteristics. A trance state is an altered somatic state that has a unique somatic profile. This somatic profile occurs entirely within the boundaries of the person's body.

Meanwhile, Deep Trance Phenomena initially occur in a specific *context*—an environment external to the person, that itself has specific environmental characteristics. For example, this context or external environment might be the first time the child encounters a drunken parent alone. In response to the threat and terror of the drunken parent (the external context), the child creates a protective Deep Trance Phenomenon (the internal state). In the early stages of this pattern between child and parent, the child's internal state will fluctuate specifically when it is confronted by the father's external threat. This is the same as saying that the traumatic response is state-dependent and context-dependent. Eventually, however, as the experience is repeated, the context will become generalized so that many different stimuli in the outer world will evoke the protective Deep Trance Phenomenon. The state-dependent experience of the Deep Trance Phenomenon remains as the basis of symptomatic behavior, which runs autonomously independent of external context. The *context* of trauma initially provoked the state-dependent response of the Deep Trance Phenomena; now, the context has been generalized so that the trance functions autonomously.

The concept of trance as a state-dependent phenomenon tells us several things: that trance can be triggered by anything in the environment, that it has a life of its own, and that the specific learnings and resources of one kind of trance are available *once that same trance* is triggered, but not available to other trance states. The resources of the different Deep Trance Phenomena operate independently; that is, *autonomously operating trances only contain the learnings of that trance state. Thus learnings are trance-specific.*

For example, I can go into a "business trance" in which I am good with numbers and objective details, but in this trance people also become objectified and my heart is not open. I feel less connected, less open. In an "intimate trance," by contrast, the softness of my heart and own vulnerability are available, and the objectivity of the business trance is not. In a "spiritual trance" in which I feel free and detached, the learnings of the business trance and the intimate trance become unreachable. This is a fragmented way of living. The greater the degree of integration of Deep Trance Phenomena, the greater the ability to have all learnings and states available *at choice*. In other words, you choose the trance rather than experiencing the trance as *coming over* you. This integration occurs with the realization that you are the creator of your own experience.

Hypermnesia: A Vigilant Trance State

I hold a special fondness for the Deep Trance Phenomenon of hypermnesia, because it was one of my primary tools of survival as a child. On first glance, hypermnesia—which means "abnormally sharp memory"—appears to be the opposite of amnesia—which means "partial or total loss of memory." From a deeper perspective, however, they are really profoundly similar in that both alter the person's "normal" memory functioning. Which direction this alteration of memory takes—toward vivid recall or blanketed forgetting—probably depends on which state is more protective and more helpful for the child. As with each Deep Trance Phenomenon we have discussed, hypermnesia (and its twin amnesia) is created as a result of a series of interpersonal interactions that somehow threaten the child.

In essence, hypermnesia is created out of what I call "resisted forgetfulness." The hypermnesic is afraid of the consequences of not remembering, of not being vigilant. Of course, when you resist forgetting, you get more forgetful. Typically, hypermnesia is spawned in childhood by an inconsistent and unstable environment, so that the only way a child can maintain control is by remembering every minute detail. He develops what might be praised as a "photographic memory," but it is a use of memory based on fear and vigilance. The need to remember everything is based on a terrible fear of the consequences of forgetting even one little thing.

In my own experience, for example, my parents were extremely inconsistent in their responses. I learned to listen to and retain every word they uttered so that later I could hold them to it. This enabled me to maintain a somewhat stable environment. My parents were always astounded by my memory and would often exclaim, "My

God, I can't believe what a memory you have. You remember absolutely everything!" Although my memory also exasperated them, because it so often proved them wrong and interrupted the entire punishment sequence, it also impressed them—which fueled my use of it well into adulthood.

The negative side of hypermnesia is the mistrustful and vigilant attitude that typically underlies it. In his attempt to survive, the child/adult keeps his intrapersonal self in a state of watchful mistrust; he watches in wait for misinformation or distortions— exaggerations, oversights, deletions, or lies. He learns to interact with the world from the coiled vantage point of his uncanny ability to "see through" any encroachments. When this state of vigilance and mistrust is taken to the extreme and joined by a few other Deep Trance Phenomena, you get a full-fledged paranoid reaction. In less extremes versions, the hypermnesic person complains of being misunderstood, of being duped, of being set up, of being deceived. To the hypermnesic, the world is a lie and he must uncover the TRUTH.

A wonderfully common example of the *state-dependent* quality of trance—in this case, a trance of hypermnesia—is the college test "all-nighter." Who in college hasn't had the experience of staying up all night to cram in all the information you need to pass the test the next day. From the time you begin the intense studying until the time you complete the test, you are in an altered state of consciousness. You are in a state of arousal in which your sympathetic nervous system pumps into your body the hormones, neurotransmitters, and peptides needed to create a state of sustained alertness. An hour after leaving the lecture hall, sitting in the cafeteria relaxing with friends, you find you can't recall one answer—and everyone hoots and hollers in delight. Your sudden forgetting occurs because your physiology in the cafeteria has shifted into an entirely different state (parasympathetic relaxation). If you were suddenly put back in the testing situation, however, you would probably know the answers once again. As your body responded to the re-arousal caused by the second testing, it would produce similar physiological conditions (sympathetic nervous system arousal) that surrounded your initial testing. The fact is that learning—especially learning that takes place under stress and pressure —is a state-dependent experience.

The hypermnesic individual is in a constant trance state of

arousal comparable to the intense but very limited period of time the student spent studying during his all-nighter. In order to sustain such a focused state, tunnel vision is necessary. This tunnel vision severely constricts the hypermnesic's range of perception; whatever pertains to the person's survival is focused on to the exclusion of just about everything else. Part of what is lost in this single-pointed focus is the person's perception of his own state-of-being. Adult children of alcoholics often exhibit hypermnesia and hypervigilance because the little girl or boy who had to take care of the alcoholic father remains in this state. Adult children of alcoholics often ensure a need for continuing this hypervigilant and hypermnesic behavior by marrying a dysfunctional person who always has to be taken care of lest some "catastrophe" occurs.

Now that I've worked with my own trance of hypermnesia, I can decide when I want to make of use it. I am free to remember everything I hear in a workshop, and I am also free to forget it. I think of it like luggage: I can pick up the state of hypermnesia in order to study or listen to a lecture, and I can put it down to watch the Celtic's play. More specifically, when I attend workshops, I give myself the suggestion that it doesn't matter what I do—I can fall asleep, space out, go to the bathroom, or doodle—and I will remember whatever is important to remember.

In actual clinical practice, hypermnesia is not common. At least, few people arrive with the complaint that they remember everything. However, hypermnesia may underlie many a complaint or symptom: the inability to maintain an intimate relationship due to an overly critical temperament; the persistence of psychosomatic disorders such as ulcers, asthma, migraines, or skin disturbances (all that prolonged tension of arousal required for remembering has to go somewhere); and it may even underlie obsessive-compulsive tendencies.

Case Example

I worked with a couple whose presenting problem was an inability to tolerate one another's differences. They each described in minute detail (minute, even though I gave them a very circumscribed time period for their "unloading") what the partner did that aggravated them. They both seemed stuck in a hypermnesic loop that went in one direction only.

My first intervention was intended to bring immediate relief to this obsessive, critical pattern by utilizing the very hypermnesia that was causing it. There was one thing they had obviously forgotten, even as they remembered each and every minor and major grievance: they had forgotten how much they loved each other. I began teasing out of them descriptions of the moment they fell in love with one another. What were they wearing? Where were they? How did their first touch feel? Their first kiss? Their first intimate lovemaking?

In this case, I was utilizing their existing hypermnesic trance abilities to retrieve resources into the present. These resources— their vividly exciting memories of their love—brought balance to their interactions as I worked with each of their symptomatic trance states.

Once you have identified the presence of a symptomatic hypermnesic trance, you can work with it by utilizing it, as I did above; or, you can work with it by suggesting the interpolation of some well-chosen amnesia as a counterbalance.

My most reliable suggestion for interpolating the experience of amnesia into the hypermnesic trance is to suggest that "You can remember only the parts of all your learnings that are relevant and important to you as an adult." You don't want the client forgetting anything useful; you don't want her to forget the injunction not to walk alone at night on the streets of New York. You *do* want her to forget the injunction imprinted on her as a child not to paint her toenails because it will make her look like a "floozy." That is a useless "learning."

Another way of offering controlled amnesia is to suggest:

> Your unconscious can begin to pick and choose among all the things that you remember. There are so many things that you no longer need, and so many things that you do need. How pleasant it is to remember unpleasant situations, realizing how much you have learned. And your conscious mind can eat the food, and your unconscious mind can digest it. Your unconscious mind already knows what it needs to keep the body fit and health, and it knows what to eliminate.

In this way, both amnesia and hypermnesia are accessed and framed in an optimal manner. Ideally, most of us make use of both amnesia and hypermnesia, depending on the circumstances. Most often, however, a struggle takes place between one set of state-dependent experiences that push us to remember and another conflicting set that push us to forget. Often, the individual has two trance identities working in opposition: one is "I have to forget what happened"; the other is, "I have to remember what happened so that it doesn't happen again." Most "seekers" are actually extremely amnesiac and are fiercely resisting the experience of amnesia. They are resisting *not knowing* by creating an identity that has to know *everything*.

Sometimes, a couple will literally embody this dichotomy. I worked with one woman who was chronically amnesic; she didn't remember anything. Her boyfriend, meanwhile, was hypermnesia. She'd tell him, "I'll be here on Friday night at 7:00 p.m.," and then would not arrive. He would get furious, accusing of her being an "inconsiderate bitch," to which she would wail, "But I never said I was going to be there. What are you talking about!" It is a dreadful merry-go-round of accusations and counter-accusations, each partner believing the other is intentionally undermining them. In reality, they are both locked in the autonomous functioning of their chosen Deep Trance Phenomenon.

Treatment of Amnesia/Hypermnesia

Amnesia

If you want to work with your own symptomatic trance state of amnesia, you can begin by using a see-saw technique:

Step One: Ask yourself, "What am I *willing* to know?" Notice whatever associations, feelings, sensations, or images arise.

Step Two: Ask yourself, "What am I *unwilling* to know?" Again, notice the inner material that surfaces.

Now, continue this questioning see-saw style, asking yourself, "What am I willing to know? What am I unwilling to know?" Take your time, being attentive to your breathing and muscle tonicity.

With an incest survivor who had no clear memories, my questions to break up the amnesic trance were as follows:

"In relation to incest, what are you willing to remember?"

"In relation to incest, what are you unwilling to remember?"

These two questions stimulate the client to remember what was forgotten.

The questions could also be phrased as:

"In relation to incest, what did you *decide* to remember?"

"In relation to incest, what did you *decide* to *not* remember?"

Repeating the questions again and again not only allows the client to remember; more importantly, the phrasing gives the client the opportunity to experience that he or she *decided* what to remember and what to forget.

Hypermnesia

The same approach can be used when working with a symptomatic trance state of hypermnesia.

Step One: Ask yourself, "What am I willing to forget?" Notice whatever associations, feelings, sensations, or images arise.

Step Two: Ask yourself, "What am I unwilling to forget?" Again, notice the inner material that surfaces.

Now, continue this questioning see-saw style, asking yourself, "What am I willing to forget? What am I unwilling to forget?" Take your time, being attentive to your breathing and muscle tonicity.

In conclusion, remembering and forgetting are *decisions* that are made and then put on automatic in a specific trance state. The decision not to remember an incest event might have been valuable for a child's survival. However, the adult who wants to complete the experience and move past it must acknowledge that the state which is inhibiting her in *present time* is the product of a past decision. Once the automatic decisions and trances are released, the resources that were being utilized to block, repress, and *not remember* automatically become available.

12

Negative Hallucination

WE HAVE ALL felt unheard, felt invisible, felt numb or bodiless at various times in our lives. Most of us were unaware that we were experiencing a Deep Trance Phenomenon called "negative hallucination." *Negative* is not a value judgment, here. It simply means *not*: *not* seeing something that is there, *not* hearing something being said directly to you, *not* feeling your own upset stomach. This does not mean that we literally stop seeing and become blind or deaf or numb on a physical, sensory level. Rather, *negative hallucination is a complex internal trance process that alters our inner experience of perception.*

Negative hallucinations come in three varieties: visual, auditory, and kinesthetic. Everyday, non-pathological examples of negative hallucination abound. With negative visual hallucination, I'm sitting at my cluttered desk, looking for the stapler, and cannot find it, even though it is sitting in plain sight. At the market, scanning rows of items, I scan right over the area I'm looking for (never mind the specific item!). Auditorially, I'm watching a Celtic's game and don't hear my wife telling me the phone is for me, even though she is standing five feet away. Kinesthetically, I discover that I've been sitting in a uncomfortably crooked position for the past half hour, but I hadn't noticed because the basketball game claimed all my focus.

Clinical examples include the husband who doesn't see that his wife is having an affair, even though the entire community knows about it. Through negative hallucination, he is able to *not* perceive all the visual, auditory, and kinesthetic cues that would reveal his wife's behavior. Auditorially, a wife will "pour her heart out" to her spouse, finally telling him how she feels—but he hears almost none of it. It is as if she were speaking Chinese. In couples therapy there is the classic example of the wife repeatedly asking her husband for more affection. Each time the issue is raised, he nods his head in assent—but nothing changes. When the problem finally reaches a crisis, the husband responds with a befuddled look as the wife gasps out, "But I told you 15 times—sitting right here in this office—I told you 15 times I needed more affection." His response: "What are you talking about? I never heard you say that. [To the therapist] Did she really say that??"

Negative hallucination is the "grand dame" of Deep Trance Phenomena, because it contains elements of *all* Deep Trance Phenomena. It, like the others, was developed to protect, support, and maintain the integrity of the child in relation to his or her familial environment (context dependent). Problems arise as this trance state begins to function autonomously (context independent), wiping out or negating varying aspects of the adult's life experience. This autonomous functioning of the trance limits the possibility of more positive experiences and creates unpleasant behavioral outcomes in the person's life. The "old habit" of not seeing, not hearing, and/or not feeling is so powerful that the individual can no longer understand his confusion and pain, which is repeatedly re-enacted in interpersonal relationships.

Negative Visual Hallucination

Our abilities to *not see* are far more extensive than most of us realize. I have worked with clients who did not know that both parents were alcoholic until they were in their thirties—even though these parents had passed out on the living-room floor countless times. The "kids" just didn't see it and had successfully blocked it from their inner recognition for over three decades.

The multitude of groups for co-dependent addictive behaviors is bringing to light the astounding degree of denial that exists. In the previous chapter, I presented the idea that the Deep Trance Phenomenon of amnesia was an old-fashioned hypnotic name for *denial*—which forms the hub of co-dependent behavior. In addition to amnesia, an individual's creation of denial will usually include one or two other trance states; most commonly, these are dissociation, confusion, and negative visual hallucination.

Every addictive person I've worked with maintains a negative hallucination for a great portion of the outer world. In order for the symptom of addiction to endure, the person has to fog out (or blank out) some portion of the outer world. In Chapter 3, I described the alcoholic woman who, in order to create the distance she had needed to survive as a child, had to *not see* much of her immediate external environment. She learned to block out the sight and sounds of fighting between her mother and father; and, most of all, she learned to blot out the sight of her father drinking and then passing out. In order to do this, she learned how to move out of the interpersonal context of sitting in the den with her father as he drank and ranted and raved, and she learned to move into the sanctuary of her self-created intrapersonal trance. The final piece to this puzzle is that the existence of the intrapersonal trance is intimately tied to her internalization of her father. Her drinking father now exists within her psyche, and the childhood conflict of "child watching father drink" is re-enacted in the adult watching herself drink. To cope with this conflict, she reproduces the same trance response in present time as she did in the past. First, she age-regresses (moves from a self-to-other trance of adult interaction into the self-to-self trance of the hurt child) and then, essentially, she *stops seeing* (negatively hallucinates) her external environment.

Whenever you encounter a *have to*—I have to work every single day, I have to have wine with my dinner, I have to exercise six times a week, I have to read at least three books a week—look for a Deep Trance Phenomenon. Addictive behavior comes in a multitude of guises, but it has one common denominator: the narrowing and fixating of attention. Negative hallucination is a *sine qua non* of trance.

Negative hallucination plays an important part in other trance experiences as well. For example, in age regression you cut yourself off from the interpersonal context and create an intrapersonal self-to-self trance. This means that you're not going to be "present" in the current year; you're going to be present "back then." Usually, to accomplish such a complex internal time-travel, a slight film will descend over your eyes; and now you are no longer watching the "film" of 1991, you're watching a "film" of a childhood replay. Likewise, in pseudo-orientation in time you also have to negatively hallucinate in order to *not see* the present but rather the future.

Negative Kinesthetic Hallucination

Negative kinesthetic hallucination (NKH) is less common than the auditory and visual varieties. Usually, NKH occurs as an offshoot of physical and/or sexual abuse. Reaction formation and interpretive distortion join forces to synthesize a subtle form of NKH. In the case of child abuse, the child initially experiences the abuse as pain. As the experience is repeated again and again, the child blocks out the sensations of pain (negatively hallucinates) and begins to interpret the experience in pleasurable terms.

I observed the case of man who was in his early thirties and very concerned about his sado-masochistic tendencies. It turned out that his father, who was a minister of "the Church," used to bring his young son down the stairs into the basement, make him pull down his pants, and proceed to hit him with a small whip or paddle. The spankings were never severe enough to draw blood or leave noticeable bruising, so this "ritual" was repeated several times a week for many years. At first, the child experienced the spankings without the intervention of any defense mechanisms—and pain was the chief ingredient. Over time, he learned to blot out the sensation of pain and take on the pleasure he unconsciously perceived his father experiencing during the spankings. Normally, when a parent spanks a child, there are visual and verbal cues that tell the child the parent does not like doing it. In this particular case, the child being spanked was confronted with cues indicating pleasure—even sexual pleasure from his father. Somehow that information was transmitted to the child; the child, in an attempt to survive this repeated trauma and minimize his discomfort, stopped perceiving the sensations as physically painful (NKH) and reinterpreted or renamed them as pleasurable. After all, pleasure is what his father was mirroring back to him throughout each episode. His father's behavior formed the context that cued the child to do likewise. It is not the least surprising that sado-masochistic sexual behavior would emerge in an adult with such a pattern in his past.

Let me stress that symptoms such as sado-masochistic behavior are the byproduct of complex psychodynamics and trance-dynamics. It is not a cleanly defined, "dot-to-dot" process of tracking Deep Trance Phenomena. The trances overlap, interweave, and coalesce. Your goal as a therapist is to discern the type of Deep Trance Phenomenon(a) that is holding the symptom together. To make this discernment, you need to diffuse focus, your in a no-trance state and, in turn, notice those Deep Trance Phenomena which seem to *direct and predominate* a patient's symptomatology.

Future Research?

The relationship between Deep Trance Phenomena and physical symptoms would be an interesting one to investigate. How correlated are our symptoms with the trances we create to protect ourselves? Do near-sighted people have a trance pattern of negative visual hallucination? I know from clinical observation that we all have proclivities that veer us toward one or two Deep Trance Phenomenon more habitually than the others. But will these trance preferences than be paralleled by clear-cut physical manifestations as well? Certainly, in my own case, the correlation exists. I was going blind until the age of 19 due to a corneal disease. And, my most used Deep Trance Phenomenon was negative visual hallucination. Perhaps it is a question that could be pursued by a graduate student in search of a thesis or dissertation topic. The implications would justify the investigation: working with Deep Trance Phenomena could be a way of preventing physical symptoms from manifesting, or certainly slowing down the disease process.

Oppositional Trances: Adding and Subtracting Reality

In Chapter 9 I introduced the concept of the *oppositional trance* and discussed it in two different contexts: one was the therapeutic use of suggesting an oppositional trance experience to a person habitually locked into, say, a pattern of dissociation; the other was the manifestation of oppositional trances in two partners. A third context for this concept exists entirely *intrapersonally*: two oppositional trance states function *simultaneously* within one person. Oppositional trance states are surprisingly common within the Deep Trance Phenomenon of negative hallucination, so that both negative *and* positive hallucination will co-exist, side-by-side, re-writing reality. In fact, in the abuse example above, the second part of the story involves the positive hallucination of pleasure after the pain has been blocked by negative hallucination.

I had a client who, after describing his "shameful" addictive behavior, said to me, "I know you're judging me—I know you think I'm weak." In fact, I was in a neutral position of observing and gathering information. In this case, the client was using both negative and positive auditory hallucinations: He was hearing things I *wasn't* saying, and he wasn't hearing what I *was* saying. The person who cannot accept compliments, who fidgets and squirms as if you're actually saying something critical to him, is often making use of this dyadic trance phenomenon of simultaneous negative and positive hallucinations. This is also true for the person with the chronic "chip on the shoulder." How does he consistently manage to re-invent the world to his detriment? By sustaining simultaneous trance states that allow him to wipe out the portion that disagrees with his position while inserting his own scripted version.

Another, graver example of oppositional trances of hallucination can be found in anorexia-bulimia: the person looks in the mirror and sees a fat body that isn't there (positive hallucination), and fails to see the rake-thin body that *is* there (negative hallucination). In Chapter 3 we discussed an example of anorexia-bulimia which was dominated by the Deep Trance Phenomenon of posthypnotic suggestion. Each person with the same symptom will be unique. If a person is more visually oriented, they might be more inclined to make use of negative and positive visual hallucinations in shaping their eating disorder.

Sexual and/or physical abuse often require extreme measures— and the co-existence of negative and positive hallucinations can often measure up to the challenge. I worked with two women, both of whom began therapy with complaints about their sexual performance: one was a premature ejaculator and the other was pre-orgasmic. The woman who "came too quickly" had a past in which her stepfather "got a kick" out of turning her on; she had to have an orgasm before he would stop. Naturally, she developed a phenomenal ability to coerce her body into rapid, orgasmic response. The responses, however, left her feeling unfulfilled.

The other woman was also sexually abused, but her abuser was totally focused on his own orgasm. She rode it out each time, trying not to feel, not to see, not to hear what was going on. To survive, she learned to freeze her body sensations and her perceptual processes.

As adults engaging in consenting sex, these women did not expect to be recreating their coping responses from the early traumas—yet they were. The trances created during childhood sexual abuse were functioning autonomously within them and consistently re-creating the past. Having sex with their partners triggered the oppositional trance states of negative and positive hallucination: they did not truly see their partner in bed with them; instead, unconsciously and unknowingly, they "saw" their past abusers; they recreated the context of the abusive stepfather, the abusive uncle, in present time.

Treatment of Negative Hallucination

In working therapeutically with yourself or with a person who habitually negatively hallucinates, ask the question: "By not perceiving what is there in the interpersonal context, how are you creating your symptomatology?" This question is one way to begin the process of *differentiation*, which forms the cornerstone of all our work with Deep Trance Phenomena. In any negative hallucination, there is a massive fog or cloud or veil of some kind that separates the person from the present interpersonal context and moves him to a past intrapersonal trance. Differentiating the symptomatic trance simultaneously initiates an expansion in the focus of attention. By offering suggestions which vary its structure, it becomes possible to take charge of its comings and goings. This "take-over" moves the trance off "automatic pilot" and relocates it as a conscious, self-generated response. By breaking out of the habitual trance patterns, you do not destroy your capacity to experience trance; you simply put it back under your own command.

Step 1: Invite the negative hallucination to reach its full potential. With whatever Deep Trance Phenomenon emerges, your first response should be to simply *allow* it to be there—totally, completely, and without judgment. As a therapist, I accomplish this by saying something to the effect of: "As you breathe and look at me, continue to just let that sense of fogginess be there. . .let it be there. . .breathe into it. . .watch it. . .feel it. . .describe that sense of fogginess as you leave a small peephole through which you breathe and look at me." I want the client to be able to experience trance with me rather than without me. This demonstrates experientially that he or she can have the trance *and* remain in an interpersonal context at the same time.

Working alone, I would sit quietly with eyes open, staring with diffused focus, and allow my vision to blur. I would spend some time just sitting with the sensation of blurred vision without doing anything to it or about it. Whenever you simply allow yourself to experience your trance in present time, you are taking charge of something that previously functioned completely autonomously.

Step 2: Expand the experience of the negative hallucination. Most of us are accustomed to our trances; consciously and/or unconsciously, we know how far they go, so to speak. I was accustomed to a certain experience of negative visual hallucination, because it was the experience that happened habitually and autonomously within me. The same is true for most people. Now, in Step 2, you go beyond this well-established border by expanding the experience. As a therapist I might say: "Now as you continue to breathe and look at me, let that fogginess grow denser. . .thicker. . .darker." Working with myself, I would make a similar suggestion internally.

Step 3: Alter the structure of the negative hallucination. Now for the fun. Take the negative hallucination as you are experiencing it in its expanded form and see if you can move it around, change its shape, size, texture, temperature, color, smell. Is it translucent or opaque? Thick or ethereal? Brightly colored, drably colored? Is it damp, sticky, or dry? Ironically, whenever you alter the structure of a negative hallucination, you are usually *adding to it.* The fog, which begins as a drab gray and neutralizes your visual experience, now evolves into a variety of sensory experiences that you "see" with vividness and clarity. This is part of the process of breaking out of the pattern of not seeing.

One specific approach I created—the "Checkerboard Technique"—provides the person with a very definite structure. Sometimes, the sense of massive *un*differentiation is so great that the person, in a sense, freezes and is unable to do anything with the trance. At that point, you can suggest that the negative hallucination is divided into four quadrants, just like a checkerboard. Then begin by asking very simple questions such as, "Which quadrant is darkest?", or by giving a suggestion: "I don't know exactly which one you'll find to be the darkest. . .It might be the upper left quadrant. . .maybe the lower left. . .perhaps the lower right. . .but, whichever, you can let me know exactly which one is darkest."

This approach instantly requires that we focus on our trance and even cut it up into smaller parts. From an undifferentiated mass, it moves into a differentiated mass with various parts and textures—which means that it is experienced differently.

Step 4: *Turnabout*. For a change of pace, give the suggestion to your client or yourself to "see what is *not* there"—in other words, begin developing the ability to experience positive hallucinations. This will give you an entirely different sensory experience from the habitual one you are accustomed to in your pattern of negative hallucination. It will also automatically stimulate resources formerly not retrievable.

Step 5: *Expand the paradox of seeing what is not seen*. You can also experiment with the question: "What else are you *not* seeing that *is* there?" Take any situation in which you have experienced yourself creating the trance of negative hallucination. In working alone with yourself, sit quietly and follow your breath as you re-create your experience of negative hallucination. Then, ask yourself the question, continue to breathe rhythmically, and watch as your mind's eye begins to scan its internal pictures.

If you are working with a client, you can verbalize a variety of possibilities as the client breathes and looks at you:

"And what else are you not seeing that is there? Perhaps you're not noticing the cat curled up on the couch. . .Maybe you're not seeing the picture on the wall near the fireplace. . .I'm not really sure. And you're probably not seeing that window at the far end of the room, or maybe it's two or three windows you're not seeing. . .I'm not really sure. And did you overlook the pile of newspapers in the corner? And are you forgetting to notice the carpeting, and the color of the paint on the walls? Or maybe there's something that you're not exactly sure what you're not seeing."

This type of trance talk automatically expands the person's focus of attention—and this expansion, in turn, releases a range of inner resources that were formerly not retrievable. When the negative hallucination is tied into early childhood trauma, a looping is established whereby the child's perception of the traumatizing parent and the child's defending Deep Trance Phenomenon become completely interlocked. The child first had to see the parental abuse in order to create negative hallucination in order *not* to see it. This looping process is part of what creates the persistent self-destructive patterns so characteristic of abused adults: They repeatedly veer toward partners who continue to embody the original trauma they are trying not to see in order to reinforce the negative hallucination that protects them!

Few clients will arrive on your doorstep with the announcement that their parents were alcoholic and they negatively hallucinate to defend against feeling that trauma. Instead the client might haltingly express some concern that her husband is drinking too much—but that she isn't sure about it, she's rather "fuzzy" about whether he is or isn't, but she has this nagging worry.

Case Example

I worked with one woman who presented in this manner. I asked her to breathe and look at me as she re-created that sensation of fuzziness; she age-regressed and slipped further into her trance of negative hallucination. I began differentiating the trance, as described above. In the next session, she returned stating: "I got angry at my husband the other day. I realized that he was drinking every day of the week, and I told him to cut it out."

The first session's work had apparently triggered the resources of increased vision and *anger*. Once the woman began to see things more clearly, her own response of anger was allowed to surface. Within a few more sessions, she was retrieving quite vivid visual memories of her alcoholic parents. As a child, she had created a fictitious boundary of defense called "negative hallucination." Now, the anger becomes a way of pushing on that boundary. The pictures of her parents in drunken stupors were not available because the negative hallucination kept the resource of anger unavailable. Once that habitual trance state is differentiated, all kinds of resources (in addition to the first one of anger) will arise naturally.

This is not to suggest that resolving a trance of negative hallucination automatically resolves all the issues around early abuse. It is simply the first layer. Once the trance is differentiated, allowing the resource of anger to float to the surface, then the client will move to another set of responses. She might, as my client did, promptly leave her spouse, declaring "I'll never have another relationship again." Now she has moved into a victim trance, so you begin to identify and differentiate the Deep Trance Phenomena that comprise the victim state.

In the first trance, the experience was, in essence:

> "I don't know my partner is drinking."
> "I'm helpless."
> "No one's good for me."

After differentiation the experience has shifted to:

> "I'm angry because he's drinking too much."
> "What am *I* going to do?"

Notice that prior to differentiation of the negative hallucination, there is an age-regressed and powerless little girl (victim). After the differentiation, she feels her own power in the form of anger and then decides to take responsibility for *her* next step.

In the next chapter, we will explore the flip side to negative hallucination, positive hallucination, and begin to get a sense of how these two Deep Trance Phenomena co-exist in the enterprise of literally re-visioning reality.

13

Positive Hallucination

LIKE ITS SISTER-TRANCE of negative hallucination, positive hallucination is not about good or bad—it is about seeing, hearing, or feeling something that is *not* there. Positive hallucinations, in their extreme form, are those strange occurrences that readily label a person "psychotic." Because we are familiar with it only its more bizarre manifestation, most of us would assume that we do not experience the Deep Trance Phenomenon of positive hallucination.

Some of the fondest "seeds" of positive hallucination are sown in childhood in the form of an imaginary friend. Some imaginary friends are quite transitory and sporadic, while others are at the child's side day and night. Hallucinatory trances will generally increase in proportion to the need to compensate for deprivation or to intensify conditions already present. For example, a child left alone once in a while might develop an imaginary friend to compensate for her feelings of isolation. However, the imaginary friend is *context-dependent* and disappears when the child encounters family members. If a child is left alone regularly and for long periods of the time, the imaginary friend might be present on an ongoing basis until the child's situation changes. In cases of abuse the child might continue to create imaginary friends well into adulthood. As with all Deep Trance Phenomena, the trance of positive hallucination is created by the child to protect her from developmental, familial, and environmental strains and traumas.

Positive hallucinations occur along a continuum in which, typically, the more vivid the hallucination, the more vivid and entrenched the underlying trauma. On the benign end of the continuum is the common experience of fantasizing: we imagine ourselves in a relationship with a particular person, we imagine ourselves learning how to high dive or skiing down an Aspen slope. Fantasizing is a normal part of our imaginative processes and remains helpful to us as along as we can create the fantasy at will and *stop* creating the fantasy at will—as long we can pick it up and put it down, so to speak. The moment the fantasy process gains periods of autonomous functioning, it moves onto the problematic portion of the hallucination continuum and becomes context-independent.

Patterns of positive hallucination become a problem when they function autonomously as defense against trauma. The less severe the history of trauma, the less intrusive the hallucination. For example, a person raised by verbally critical (as opposed to physically abusive) parents might have a mildly paranoid response whenever he is in a group situation, imagining (hallucinating) that someone "over there" is making a critical or snide remark about him. Toward the more extreme end of the continuum, we find the case of the woman mentioned previously who believed "beings" were actually speaking to her, preparing her to be Christ's successor. This woman's home-life had been intolerable as a child, so, as discussed in Chapter 8, she had used pseudo-orientation in time to project herself into a better future, and she had used positive hallucinations to create a specific and (to her perception) tangible "content" to that future. Now, as an adult confronted by a dreary re-enactment of her caretaker role, she used age regression to return to the childhood state in which the positive hallucinations had first emerged. Typically in issues of co-dependency there is so much age regression and positive hallucination that the adult child is continually reliving the past in present time. This is why so many co-dependent people find it difficult to leave a spouse; they fear for their lives, or believe they cannot take care of themselves—responses that are a product of Deep Trance Phenomena.

Many of our overly sensitive reactions involve positive hallucinations—pictures or voices of past experiences that we super-impose over the present moment. Who hasn't had the experience of being absolutely devastated by criticism from a boss or superior? The *real* situation in the present moment is that the boss has found some inadequacies in your report that need to be rectified. The situation in the *hallucinated* version is that you are a total failure who is going to lose his livelihood in the next five minutes. Given that the boss is *not* standing there and telling you that you are worthless, from what source does this version come? It comes from a "pop-up" of an automatic trance that includes age regression and positive hallucination.

People who are well-entrenched in a "victim mentality" make vigorous use of positive hallucination. The person with the prover-bial "chip on his shoulder" is carrying around the Deep Trance Phenomenon of positive hallucination, sprinkling it across all the interactions of his day. Without it, the present moment would be just that—unfettered by the constant list of gripes and injustices. Adults who are victims of traumas such as rape or assault will usually find themselves, wittingly or unwittingly, plagued by positive hallucinations of their assailant. Walking down a street in broad daylight is no longer a mundane experience for the woman who was raped at three o'clock in the afternoon. Now she is continually "seeing" her assailant at every turn. Positive hallucinations also can take the form of age-regressed flashbacks in cases of post-traumatic stress experienced by rape and incest victims as well as war veterans.

Oppositional Trances

As mentioned in the previous chapter, in many cases *two* oppositional trance states are required to restructure reality: nega-tive hallucinations are used to eradicate any portions of reality that disagree with what the individual needs to create; and positive hallucinations are used to construct the "corrected" version. Simul-taneous hallucinations are rampant in interpersonal communications and in intimate relationships:

> A man and woman are having their first date. The man says, "You look nice." The woman thinks: "He wants to have sex with me."

A man approaches a woman at a party, smiles, and inquires, "How are you?" The women returns a guarded look while concluding to herself: He is coming on to me.

A man and a woman have been conversing during a break at a conference. The woman says, "I'd like to have lunch with you." The man thinks, "Oh-oh, she wants to have a relationship with me."

Instead of hearing a simple compliment, a simple question, a simple luncheon invitation, the other person "hears" (and is threatened by) an entirely different script. Perhaps this phenomenon of interfacing trance experiences is at the root of the problem we describe as "being on different wavelengths." The two simultaneously functioning trances cancel out the possibility of clear reception of either trance communication.

Along far more serious lines is the experience of abuse, which often triggers oppositional trances of negative and positive hallucinations. These twin trances work to (1) blot out the painful, real-life experience and (2) invent, construct, create a tolerable, hallucinatory one. Learning to label pain as pleasure cannot occur without the pivotal co-creations of simultaneous Deep Trance Phenomena.

The Therapeutic Utilization of Positive Hallucinations

As a therapist, I often encourage myself to drop into a trance as I breathe and watch the client. This trance might include positive hallucinations from which I derive metaphors or new understandings for myself of what is taking place. Some might call this "intuition" rather than hallucination. In my experience, both can fall along the same continuum of accessing information—but in the case of positive hallucinations, there is an unusually vivid visual component.

One afternoon I was working with a client who complained that he had problems making changes. As I listened to him and observed him, I went into a trance with my eyes open and "saw" him making love to his wife. I immediately utilized the "information" in the hallucinated images to access common everyday experiences of making changes as the basis for a series of suggestions:

"When you're making love with your wife, you can. . .change positions and still feel very comfortable. You might. . .want her to move there, or you to move here, or this to move, or that to move. And even as you make all those *changes* throughout all of your lovemaking, you still can. . .continue to feel comfortable. . . .And I don't have to tell you that you can. . .make *change* for somebody out of your pocket or you can. . .*change* your clothes and not even know that you're doing it—and isn't it nice to know you can. . .make these *changes*."

Where did the image come from? Was I tapping into "psychic" areas? Was *I* simply caught by my own projection? My only answer is that I chose to go into a trance state and in some way join or unite with or cooperate with my client's trance state. We create a mutual trance state which fosters an unconscious-to-unconscious connection—rather than the conscious-to-conscious connection that typifies more traditional therapies. Erickson and Rossi talk about "depotentiating the conscious mind" of the patient to facilitate trance; I followed that same principle, only with myself as the therapist. By depotentiating my own conscious mind set, the availability of all my unconscious perceptual resources is widened and deepened considerably. By choosing to go into trance as the therapist, I create the possibility for *looping*, whereby the client's unconscious processes loop into my unconscious processes, and in a sense, there no longer are two people in the room—but one.

In a session with another client who was alcoholic and wanted to have a baby, at one point I looked at her and saw a baby with pajamas like Dr. Denton's—except, the baby was actually a bottle of booze. I gave her the assignment to continue her drinking, but to put the bottle inside a pair of baby pajamas. She was unable to drink! The jarring sight of the baby pajamas holding her alcohol exaggerated her relationship to alcohol as being, symbolically, her unborn, wished-for baby. She couldn't have a baby because she was already monogamous with alcohol—she already had a "baby" called Alcohol. The choice point was so compelling, she was able to discontinue drinking.

Carl Whitaker (1989) allows himself to fall asleep during therapy! While he naps, he invariably dreams something that is pertinent to the client. Sleeping and hallucinating may seem at opposite ends of the experiential continuum, but as therapeutic techniques they are really quite related: both are altered states of consciousness incorporating a vivid visual component that communicates information unavailable in the normal waking state. One of Whitaker's most valuable legacies to therapists is his own learning to trust *whatever* he experiences as a therapist. If hallucinating is a natural trance experience for you, than you may find many creative ways to make use of it in sessions.

Projections as Hallucinations

The psychodynamic process of projection plays a significant role in all kinds of relationships—personal, therapeutic, professional, and collective. Projection is generally thought of as an unconscious defense against repressed material about oneself that is projected upon another. I prefer to view projection as part of the Deep Trance Phenomenon of positive hallucination. In the therapy setting, positive hallucination produces the experience we label "transference/countertransference." The client looks at me and sees Daddy. I look at the client and see my mother. We are both seeing what is *not* there. Transference and countertransference are, in essence, trance states that make use of positive hallucination and age regression.

In working with a client who is projecting someone else onto me, I begin by having him pick out some aspect of my appearance that stands out: my beard, my glasses, a ring on my finger, whatever. In a trance which includes the client's projection/hallucination, I acknowledge the projection and then structure the task that will differentiate me from the projected person: "I remind you of your father? I didn't realize I was that old. I wonder, could you look at me and pick out something I am wearing that attracts your attention?" The client picks something and then I instruct him: "Whenever you imagine that I am like your father, I would like you to. . .look at my beard. . .look at my ring finger"—whatever has been selected. This simple technique differentiates me from the client's context and helps re-focus him in the present moment.

Another approach I use is a Gestalt technique I learned in the mid-seventies from Eric Marcus, M.D. In this approach I place a chair in the center of the room and ask the client to hallucinate an image of his father sitting in it. I would place my chair next to the empty chair and instruct the client to make direct eye contact with me while stating, "Stephen, this is my father and this is you. You are similar because. . ." The client would list all the reasons we were similar—all the reasons for the transference "hook." Next, I would instruct the client to continue making eye contact with me while stating, "Stephen, this is my father, and this is you. You are different because. . ." At this point the client usually froze, unable to answer, because he was still in his transference trance. Once the shift was made out of the transference trance, the client began to list many, many differences.

Sexual issues will also arise that can be treated from a similar vantage point. One woman I was working with reported having strong, obsessional sexual fantasies about me. My statement was: "When you look at my face, imagine that my face is a rubber mask that you can just take off, at will. When you take off the mask, what do you see?" She saw her brother's face—which opened a slew of traumatic memories in which she was beaten and molested by her brother. As a homework assignment, I asked her to continue to have sexual fantasies but to put her brother's face on my face (this made the implicit explicit). Secondly, I asked her to put a "brother mask" on those men about whom she obsessed. This not only made the implicit explicit, it brought the sexual abuse of her brother into focus and into present time. Furthermore, it helped to alleviate the transference of seeing me as her brother, which shifted our therapeutic relationship.

I find that this approach is simple, direct, and atheoretical. It enables the person to be with me in present time, and at the same time work through issues with the parent—without wasting months and months on elusive transference issues that, in this framework, constitute just another trance state. In handling my own so-called countertransference issues, I take the simple route of observing what is occurring, knowing that I am creating a projection trance, and continue my work. I find it quite natural to be attracted to an interesting person and would be surprised if I weren't. In my thinking, it is somewhat paradoxical that so much fuss is made over so-called transference-countertransference issues, given the nature of the traditional therapeutic encounter. Therapists have historically tended to create the therapy room as though it were a make-believe world. A client is seated or asked to lie on a couch while talking or "free associating," and the therapist hides behind his/her role (and sometimes even his/her desk) as all-knower and makes brilliant observations. Naturally the client is going to relate to the therapist as though he were his father! The more real *we* get as therapists—the less ensconced in the role we allow ourselves to be—the less transference/countertransference.

Treatment of Positive Hallucination

1. *Identifying what is there*. Since positive hallucination involves the perception of some kind of stimuli that are *not* present, a simple way to begin interrupting this particular trance is to ask yourself/your client to see what *is* there: identify the furniture in the room; consciously notice the environmental sounds; take note of exactly how you are interacting, sensorially, with the bed, chair, couch, or floor with which you are in contact. This will enhance your focus of awareness and automatically alter your subjective experience.

2. *Owning the hallucination*. Begin by recognizing the positive hallucination as part of the client's or your own experience. It is part of you/them, it helped you as a child, it may even help you as an adult. Acknowledge the integral role this Deep Trance Phenomenon has played in your life. Meditate on the question, "How can I *own* this part of myself?" Try *pretending* to own the hallucination—be the voice, image, or sensation. See/feel/hear it as part of your own inner fabric. Re-integrate the hallucination as a part of yourself.

Example: The woman who was hallucinating "beings" was asked to *pretend* that the beings who came to see her were actually coming from *inside* her. I asked, "How would you feel pretending this is true, right now, in this room?" She responded with immediate relief and was comfortably able to "pretend" the hallucinations were being generated by *her*.

Much is implied in this woman's owning of her own hallucinations. An important part of this woman that is not integrated—or even acknowledged—is that part that wants to be admired. If I were to make the direct statement to her, "You really want to be admired, don't you?", she would answer, aghast, "No, I don't!" Her need to be admired is disowned, just as the hallucinations are disowned. She needs to re-integrate that part of herself which is dissociated and which contains the dissociated resource of admiration.

3. *Re-create the hallucination repeatedly.* Give yourself/your client the task of creating the hallucination in a variety of different ways. Each time, you will gain a deeper sense of *yourself as creator* rather than as victim of a process you cannot control. Create the hallucination; cease to create it. Re-create it again, looking/sounding/feeling a bit different; cease to create it. In relation to the positive hallucination, let yourself experience the sense of "picking it up and putting it down," as though it were an actual object. This is very much a technique of paradoxical therapy: if you intentionally or purposefully create in present time something that has functioned autonomously within you, then you have taken charge of "it."

3. *Differentiate the hallucination.* Now give yourself the experience of sustaining the hallucination while altering it. Enlarge it, shrink it, move it around, give it a rhythm, give it a sound or texture, frame it, float it, color it. This reinforces the experience of yourself as creator.

Example: A woman came to see me complaining that she always heard her mother's voice inside her mind. As an assignment I suggested that she spend about 20 minutes each evening imagining a record of her mother's voice playing at a speed of 45 rpm. She was then instructed to alternate the speed from 45 rpm to 78 rpm back down to 33 rpm. In addition, she was to alternate the sound as it came out of each stereo speaker by regulating the balance, treble, and bass. By carrying out this assignment for one week, she was able to gain control over voices that had plagued her for two decades. When I asked her what she would call the record, she replied, "Mom's Greatest Hits."

14

Confusion

IN THIS CULTURE we are taught to "break through" or "get clear of" our confusion. The label, "Confusion is bad," is deeply embedded in our collective psyche. Our resistance to experiencing the experience of confusion, along with the "bad" label, keep this trance frozen in time.

Although most of us are not accustomed to thinking of confusion as an actual trance, it is both a Deep Trance Phenomenon in its own right as well as the pivotal bridging mechanism in the creation of hypnotic identities. As we shall see later, confusion is the transitional state in which a person shifts out of his real self and into the creation of defensive or compensatory identities. In order to "get clear," the person resists his initial trance of confusion by creating a part of himself—an identity—whose goal is to "get clear."

Erickson was probably the first hypnotherapist to recognize the trance qualities of confusion and make use of them to induce therapeutic trance in his patients. In my approach confusion is not induced by the therapist—it is brought in by the client. As with all other Deep Trance Phenomena, I do not impose confusion on the client as a trance-inducing technique, but rather *observe the client's own creative use of confusion* as a symptomatic trance pattern of response. In such cases, confusion has been used by the individual to self-induce a trance that protects him/her from a threatening external stimulus.

Confusion is a naturalistic trance state which emerges when the child is overwhelmed by an event, interaction, or emotion. Because of the threat, the child *resists* experiencing the episode, and it is in the resisting process that a state of confusion or disorientation emerges. Once resisted, the child will protect himself from the non-experienced experience by surrounding it with confusion and creating an "identity" that can meet or stop the overwhelming stimulus. Confusion provides the shift in consciousness out of which the coping mechanisms of the new identity are selected.

Parents often make demands on children that are experienced as overwhelming, impossible, or simply unacceptable. Sometimes the demands and expectations which the child is unable to fulfill create feelings of confusion and disorientation. The confusion becomes the way in which the child handles the event, and it is also the "space" in which he creates an identity that *can* handle things.

A simple example: A young child is eating his dinner with his hands and his mother reproofs him harshly. If the child is unable to experience the threatening feeling of his mother's reprimand, and/ or if the expression of that threatening feeling is not allowed or received by the parent (*you can't say that*), then the child will abort his natural, uninhibited response. Aborting the child's ongoing response mode triggers confusion and disorientation, followed by a search for a way to respond adequately to the stimulus (Mother's anger). If this pattern becomes chronic—if the child repeatedly attempts to express himself and the parent responds with *you can't*—then eventually the child will create a major shift in himself to accommodate the *you-can't* impingement on his being. In essence, the very young child's nature is to be completely open to all things—what I call "pure being." When this pure beingness is assaulted by core messages of *you can't*, *don't*, *stop it*, confusion sets in (in computer-ese, a kind of "can't compute" response) in which the child shrinks his focus of attention from his full being to become a confused little being.

Now a fascinating process gets underway. In this "pot" of confusion within the child are the ingredients of many possible identities—those concise belief structures that appear to dissipate both the confusion and the strife. First one identity will be synthesized

out of certain ingredients, and then a second identity—an oppositional identity—will invariably follow. We have touched on this
concept of oppositional identities and will explore it in greater detail
in Chapter 19. For now, I want to emphasize the special role played
by confusion in this complex psychic chess game.

The first hypnotic identity that emerges for the child in our
above example is called "I want it my way," and its goal is the
child's autonomy of behavior. The child might try this one out first
and if it works, he will continue to use it. The moment it stops
working, he again will be thrown into a state of confusion, out of
which emerges a second identity called "I'll do anything to please
you." If, for example, Mother's messages escalate from *you can't*
to *don't talk to me like that* to *you're bad—stay in your room*, the
child might come to the conclusion that his only choice of response
to get out of the confusion of Mother's rejection is *I'll do whatever
you want me to do*. The goal of this identity is to win love, affection,
and approval.

Both identities now co-exist, side by side, creating a sustained
state of conflict and tension—a real power struggle—within the
child. To lessen the conflict, the child learns to project one identity
while owning the other. Let's say Billy projects the identity "I'll do
anything to please you," while proudly owning the identity of "I
want it may way." What pattern is Billy most likely to manifest in
school? That of the acting-out child. The projected identity is
scorned by Billy and at the same time is used by him to fuel his
stance of "I want it my way—and *you'll* do anything to please me."
In the reverse, Billy might project the identity "I want it my way"
onto all authority figures, going through life in his conscious
identity of "I'll do anything to please you." Either pattern is highly
limiting and distorting, not to mention exhausting.

More often than not, we flip-flop back and forth between our
two oppositional identities rather than remain rigidly locked into
one while steadfastly projecting the other. For example, say you are
working as a secretary in a corporation and an employee comes up
to you and starts trying to please you in order to get in to see the boss.
Since the employee is playing out "I'll do anything to please you,"
you flip into "I want it my way." In your tersest voice, you instruct
the employee to "sit over there—he'll get to you when he can."

Another day you find yourself interviewing for a promotion. As you sit across the shiny solid teak-wood desk from your interviewer, you rapidly slip into "I'll do anything to please you," while projecting "I want it my way" onto the other person. This flip-flopping phenomenon is, I believe, a key aspect of the co-dependent relationship. The co-dependent who offers the addict a drink at one point in the evening and then, hours later shouts, "Why are you drinking?", is ice-skating expertly along an inner landscape of dual oppositional identities.

When the pattern does not flip-flop, you get an individual who usually has a reputation as either a bear ("I want it my way) or a wimp ("I'll do anything to please you"). In a surprisingly fragile way, the playing out of this identity is contingent on everybody else playing out the projected identity. The moment the projected identity is not "received" out there, the person's equilibrium is disturbed and confusion rushes in. I had a client who unflinchingly sustained a "bear" identity of "I'm doing it my way and you're going to please me." If you objected that you didn't want to do it his way, he would become even more autocratic. The refusal only further intensified his owned identity. Instead of taking on his projected identity and either accepting it or refusing it, I responded with disinterest and neutrality. In essence, by my neutral behavior I said, "I don't really care if I do it your way or not." This pattern interruption invariably threw him into confusion—he had no idea what to do once the black-and-white polarity of the oppositional identities had been stripped away. Without the polarity, with only shades of gray left, he had no blueprint for his behavior.

The above example is obviously a simplification and/or condensation of a very complicated process. Yet the bare bones of this structure whereby oppositional identities are created out of confusion is quite valid and useful. It is also important to remember that the same event experienced by two different children will net two different trance responses. Another child might respond to her mother's harsh reprimand by throwing up a trance of negative auditory hallucination or dissociation rather than confusion.

The Contexts of Confusion

Every confusion trance during childhood begins its life, so to speak, in a context of circumstances. This context will fall into one of three general categories: task/objects, interpersonal, or self-generative. That is to say, the confusion will happen in response to a task or object, an interpersonal interaction, or be generated by the child herself.

I. *Task and Object-Oriented Confusion.* In this first variety of the confusion trance, objects and our ability to manipulate them become the pivot-point of confusion and anxiety. Say the parent expects the three-year-old child to make a peanut-butter-and-jelly sandwich by herself. She attempts to do so, but spills things, tears the bread, and winds up crying. Mother remonstrates her, saying that she's old enough to know how to make a sandwich for herself. Each time this pattern is repeated, the little girl goes into a state confusion and is unable to accomplish the task. Out of this confusion emerges an identity called "I can't do anything right." This identity accompanies the little girl into adulthood, is generalized onto numerous tasks and objects, and is consistently fused with age regression. Confusion is placed on automatic by the child and now operates in the adult as the "solution" to *all* problems related to tasks and objects—not just in response to making sandwiches.

Another example might by the little boy who is trying to remember how to operate his new electric train and has to repeatedly ask his father for help. Dad gets exasperated and shouts, "Quit pestering me—do it yourself!" The child goes into confusion, which is paired with the electric train. A few days later, he asks his father how to make a telephone call. The father is again impatient and tells him, "Just punch the numbers." These experiences lay the groundwork for the automatic response of confusion to a wide range of objects—from electric trains and telephones, to gadgets and tools, to stereos, computers, and automobiles.

Authority figures—or holograms of them—tend to play a prominent role in this trance. The sixth-grader who is confronted with his first computer and goes into a frenzy of anxiety is re-creating his father in present time. The "hologram" of the father hovers over the child with the remonstration, "Why can't you operate the computer!"

II. *Interpersonal Confusion.* In this second type of confusion, the child learns to use confusion to manipulate the environment in a particular way. Let's take an example similar to our above one, but alter the parental response. Say the little girl, when asked to perform some task, looks up at Daddy with a confused look on her face. Daddy then shows her how to do, and in fact, handles the task in the process. Later, Mommy asks her to help with dinner, but again she gets confused and Mommy does everything for her. After several repetitions of this pattern, the little girl learns that looking, acting, or being confused results in getting someone else to do things for her. This contrasts with the above example in which the confusion brought only remonstrations. When it brings a desired outcome, it then plunks in like any other learned response. Once this identity is surrounded by amnesia and placed on automatic, it appears real and genuine and is supported and reinforced by the familial/social network.

III. *Self-Generated Confusion*. Here the child learns to *generate* confusion within the family environment as a means of protecting himself. This is a defensive creation which nets the child a subtle sense of safety and control. In essence, the child learns how to out-smart, out-maneuver his parents and the situations that overwhelm him. He learns that by using certain words, by displaying certain specialized types of knowledge or information, the adults remain bewildered and slightly out-of-control. Although it appears as though the child who is generating the confusion is not actually *in* a state of confusion himself, the opposite is true. It is the child's ongoing shifts into confusion that *require* his externalization of the confusion in a manner that *he* controls.

Overly intellectual individuals will often make use of confusion in order to present a facade of control and stability. Underneath the intellectualism—which is often daunting to others and throws them into their own defensive trance states—is a confusion-identity against which the individual is constantly defending.

I discussed another facet of this phenomenon in Chapter 11 on amnesia and hypermnesia, noting that as a child, I had made use of a hypervigilant memory to confuse and astound my parents, keeping them off guard and "off my case." Here we see how various Deep Trance Phenomena "team up" to create the desired protection or feeling. It is important to understand that trances rarely function in isolation, but rather form a dynamic, interactive network of defense.

Self-generated confusion is by no means confined to the intellectual arena. Kids who specialize in acting-out behavior are experts—even masters—of the self-generated confusion trance. I had a marvelous experience in a residential treatment facility that perfectly demonstrates a very non-intellectual use of this third type of confusion. The kids were all juveniles and all highly volatile. They would try anything to gain control over their environment. One kid found his niche by making statements that shocked the counselors. He would go up to a counselor and announce, "Your mother gives your father blow jobs." The counselor would invariably be shocked by the statement and not know how to respond—which would give the kid an illusory sense of having some control over his environment.

I had already seen this routine happen a couple of times when my turn came. The kid strutted up to me and shouted, "Your mother gives your father blow jobs!" My response was, "I hope so, because my father sure would be frustrated if she didn't." His mouth dropped open and *he* went into confusion—at which point I began to do a few minutes of therapeutic trance work with him.

Therapists and Confusion

Therapists are not supposed to get confused. At worst, they might have to admit, "I don't know the answer to that," but this not knowing is usually couched in comforting certainty. The deep need we have as therapists to "get clear" and "understand" is often, at least in part, a resistance to the experience of confusion. When a therapist is confronted by his or her own confusion and *doesn't* acknowledge it, you will get the same reactive identity formations as you do with a threatened child. There are countless variations of these, but two common ones are what I call the "smart-person identity" and the "calm, cool, and collected identity."

My suggestion to therapists—and it is a suggestion I frequently put to practice in my own therapy sessions—is to knowingly and intentionally *be confused.* Allow yourself to feel the sensations of confusion fully; look at it from a completely new vantage point of *no judgment.* It is a very novel and entertaining experience to take away the negative label and go on the assumption that confusion is as valid a response to experience as is clarity. . .understanding. . . empathy. Amazingly, the confusion paradoxically disappears rather rapidly and connection to the unconscious again becomes available in an uninterrupted flow of awareness.

Abuse and Confusion: Strange Bedfellows

Traumatic experiences of molestation and abuse always involve a complex interaction of Deep Trance Phenomena. As a therapist, where do you begin? Do you pinpoint one trance over the others? Or do you try to work with all of them?

Often in cases of abuse, the Deep Trance Phenomenon of confusion will function as the "hub" of the "trance wheel." The trance of confusion is created and thrown up, so to speak, as a buffer zone in which other Deep Trance Phenomena can be constellated. During the molest, the child goes into disorientation and confusion because the stimulus—the perpetrator—is so overwhelming that she doesn't know how to respond. In that space she creates an identity called "fear of men" that is triggered by all males. At the same time she *fuses* with the perpetrator, thus creating two oppositional identities: the victim or perpetrated person, *and* the perpetrator. The victimized child now co-exists in her psyche with Uncle Henry. As a young woman, she will project the perpetrator identity, choosing men who will act out the physical abuse. The important point to understand is that *all of this complex process takes place in the presence of confusion.*

I have used many examples of abuse and molestation to illustrate the functioning of various Deep Trance Phenomena. The trance of confusion is where the shift into hypnotic identities takes place, and thus is very important for incest/abuse survivors who invariably create identities in response to their traumatic experiences.

Treatment of Confusion

(1) *Allow yourself to feel the confusion.* The first stage of working therapeutically with the Deep Trance Phenomenon of confusion is to allow yourself to be fully confused. Treat it like an experiment in which, probably for the first time, your assignment is to welcome confusion as an interesting phenomenon. Notice any sensation, feeling, or image that comes up, allowing it full expression.

Throughout this process continue to breathe rhythmically, noting which areas of your body tighten in response to feeling confused. Then tighten those area and intentionally hold your breath, now consciously re-creating your experience of confusion. *Merge with the experience/sensation/feeling of confusion.* In this way you experience a *whole body awareness* of the confusion in present time, which automatically changes its expression.

(2) *Differentiate the confusion.* As with all Deep Trance Phenomena, the trance of confusion is experienced as an undifferentiated mass. First find an image of your undifferentiated experience of the confusion—be it a dark cloud, a block, a barricade, a fog, and so forth. Take the image and notice in detail the specific areas of the confusion, assigning a different adjective to each different area. For example: clear, dry, open, clogged, porous, translucent, dark, cloudy, smothering, cold, biting, chaotic, glacial, laser-like, and so forth. Differentiating the amorphous feeling of confusion will automatically change your subjective feeling.

3. *Witness the confusion.* Utilize the entire experience of confusion by watching or witnessing it "just as it is," with no judgment or desire to remove it. In a sense, you take your awareness out to the edges of the confusion experience and observe it. Note that this approach differs from the first one in which you allowed yourself to *merge* with the experience of confusion. Now, you are going to simply watch it, and to do that, you will naturally expand your awareness to the outermost edges of the confusion. By witnessing the experience of confusion, changes automatically occur and the "stuckness" diminishes.

4. *Symbolize the confusion.* Symbols or images of your own internal resources can be evoked and intermixed with the confusion trance. This intermixture automatically shifts the experience of confusion into one of clarity and comfort. This technique is particularly helpful when the confusion occurs in an interpersonal context. For example, let's say you are in an anxious state about an upcoming business lunch because of your tendency to "space out" when you are nervous, get confused, and become completely inarticulate. First, re-create these feelings in present time as you breathe rhythmically. Allow the confusion to express fully.

Once the sensation of confusion is in place, ask your unconscious for a symbol or image that can aid you in the luncheon interaction.

In your mind's eye you see a picture of a beautiful tree. Ask yourself where you want to place the symbol in your body. This step is critical because trance is experienced *in the body*. Place the image in your heart area, for example. Now feel the image in your heart and also see it in the heart of the person with whom you are to interact. Your completed image is one of two people over lunch, with two beautiful trees radiating from the heart area. The confusion trance, which threatened to usurp the meeting, is now "diluted" if not completely transformed by the energy from the symbolic inner resource. In addition, you've expanded your context of experience, as discussed in Chapter 6, on two important levels: it now includes your body (via your heart) and the larger social network (your colleague). Your context is increasingly expanded in a manner that naturally results in a therapeutic resolution of your confusion.

This method of asking for a symbolic resource can be applied in any situation you find distressful or uncomfortable. I once used it to get through a tooth-pulling. Before going to the dentist I asked my unconscious for a resource. Up popped a picture of Adolf Hitler getting his tooth pulled! As I sat in the dental chair undergoing this most dreaded procedure, I happily watched Adolf suffer through it, which helped me dissociate from the physical me who was losing the tooth.

You can cultivate a channel of communication between your conscious and unconscious minds so that any time you need assistance, you ask for a resource and remain open to receiving a response. In the midst of thrashing confusion, ask for a symbol, and notice where you can put it in your body to "ground" it.

15

Time Distortion

TIME DISTORTION interrupts our linear, temporal, sequential world in a way that has profound implications about the nature of so-called reality. For most of us, though, the profound implications have to wait in the wings as we wade through our more mundane uses and misuses of time.

Consensual reality tells us that *time* is an absolute and objective factor, yet every day we experience time in a purely *subjective* manner that often completely disobeys what we might call "clock time." Through the Deep Trance Phenomenon of time distortion, we lengthen or shorten our subjective experience of time. Time, for all human beings, is experienced *subjectively*, not objectively, and as such, it is experienced in direct accord with how we *choose* to experience our life. We are responsible, then, for how we experience the passage of time, and we can learn to alter our experience of time itself according to our individual needs and choices.

Like all Deep Trance Phenomena, time distortion as a symptomatic trance for the adult has its genesis as a protective device for a threatened or overwhelmed child. The child may look for ways to make her "happy times" last longer and to shorten the "bad times" in which mom and dad are fighting, for example. Unfortunately, there is a paradoxical reversal of the outcome: any attempt to resist experiencing an unpleasant event actually makes time feel subjectively longer. The child who is trying to make her parents' fight go by more quickly will automatically impede her somatic equilibrium by now holding her breath and tightening her muscles. The body in its tightened, held state actually *slows down the individual's subjective experience of time*; holding the breath creates a "frozen" experience that "holds" the feelings and impedes the outward flow of emotions. The fight between mom and dad feels like it lasts four hours, whereas in clock time it involved a mere ten minutes.

It appears as though time and resistance are directly correlated: the greater the resistance, the more time is experienced as moving slowly. Without resistance, time "flies by." This is another paradox of how we create our experience of time: we experience time as passing very quickly when we are enjoying ourselves. Why is this? Somatically, we are not resisting the experience—indeed, may even be welcoming the experience—and thus our muscles are loose and relaxed, our breathing, rhythmic and soothing.

The overall outcome of how we typically experience time shows us one way in which we consistently choose pain over pleasure: for most of us, painful or traumatic events in our lives remain frozen in time and appear to have lasted a very long time, creating impacts that will take an even longer period of time to "work through." Pleasurable events, meanwhile, are barely recalled and are not often recognized as having longlasting impact. Painful events are resisted and therefore appear to last longer, while pleasant ones appear to be fleeting.

Clinically, we see this imbalance almost across the board: if a person has, say, ten experiences and one of them is bad, it appears as though nine of them are bad and only one of them is good! In other words, as therapists we will encounter the Deep Trance Phenomenon of time distortion in almost every single problem a client brings us.

There is a story told by Swami Muktananda to illustrate this subjective use of time. A man and a woman are happily married for ten years. For two days in the tenth year, the man has an affair while on a business trip. The wife discovers the affair and promptly "forgets" the past ten years. The affair is now emphasized as if it were the whole story of this couple's relationship. If this woman were to come into therapy to deal with the affair, you can bet she wouldn't sit there talking about her ten years of happy marriage. All the resources, learnings, sharings, and experiences of the "pre-affair" time period will be diminished if not entirely negated. She will then spend a year or two in therapy recovering from one two-day incident. This is time distortion: the ten years of happy marriage now seem to have gone by so quickly as to virtually not have happened and to have left no impact, while the day of the discovery of the affair seems to last forever and carry all the impact.

In cases of severe family pathology and abuse, painful events will comprise a large chunk of clock time, but for many of us, past painful events appear to rule our lives even though these events may have comprised only one-twentieth of our total life experience. This is because the tightness of muscles and the holding of breath "freezes" the experience in time, in the *body*. The psychotherapy of Wilhelm Reich and its later evolution into Alexander Lowen's Bioenergetics further emphasize this point: Trance states hold trauma not only psychologically but somatically as well. Every trance state has a body component which needs to be acknowledged and processed. This is why I refer many of my clients for Rolfing or the Feldenkrais method of body work.

Even when past trauma is extensive, however, the therapeutic use of time distortion can still be quite helpful. The idea is to help the individual *lengthen* her experience of pleasurable events while *shortening* the painful ones. What you are actually doing is helping the client to experience the trauma in terms of "clock time." The paradoxical nature of time distortion is thus thwarted, as the traumatic events are recontextualized in relation to clock time. A young child who is molested once by her visiting uncle will experience the actual act of molest for an hour—yet it make take her years and years of therapy to undo that molest process. Basically, what has happened is that the event in time—the molest—becomes both the central point of focus as well as the entire context for the child's life. I am suggesting that a much quicker way of dealing with the molest is to recontextualize the trauma by helping the individual re-own the rest of her life.

One of the problems with the co-dependent groups is the fixation of identity within the pathology: "I'm an alcoholic," "I'm an incest survivor," "I'm an overeater," are *identities* that exclude large portions of the self while leaving it labeled in a very limiting way. While the original purpose of identifying oneself in this manner is quite helpful—to bring the person out of denial—the long-term result is a rigid, permanent identity of limitation and pathology. I am not negating the huge success of the co-dependent groups (modeled after Alcoholics Anonymous), but rather suggesting an area of limitation that could be altered to further enhance success.

The Time Continuum

There is a continuum of pleasure and pain along which we travel—or try to travel—throughout life. For most of us this continuum has shrunk to a very small, small area so that our range of experience lies within fairly cramped quarters. The rule that governs the pain-pleasure continuum is: The more I resist my pain, the more I resist my pleasure. The two are inextricably linked. As we continually narrow our experience of the continuum, life becomes increasingly monotonous and robot-like. A wasteland of our own resources lies on both sides of our circumscribed "plot" on the continuum.

Time distortion is the transducer that translates chronological time into our subjective experience of it. As such, it plays an important role in shrinking our experience of the life continuum— when we use it to do so. We can make just as ready use of it to reverse a subjective experience we find to be unpleasant or undesirable and to expand our range of response along the continuum.

A person who uses time distortion symptomatically often couples it with age regression to fixate experience of present time in the past trauma. The child who found herself in the threatening or unwanted situation in effect "took a picture" of what she *didn't* want to happen and continued to "hold" that picture within herself. Consequently, all else—the remaining context of her life—is viewed through the filter of this picture. Any good experience will be filtered through the resisted experience—and the resisted experience will come out ahead. Through the chronic use of time distortion as an adult, she will constantly look back to the past and project it into the future. In other words, she will always be living in trauma.

Time distortion, like any other Deep Trance Phenomenon, is a patterned, habitual response involving a shrinking of the focus of

Time Distortion ◆ 179

attention and a concomitant diminution of the person's experiential context. How we experience time in the present is shaped by where we focus our attention in the past. However, if attention can be narrowed and fixated, it can also be expanded and made fluid. You begin by getting a sense of how the person holds the past in present time; where the person falls along the continuum of past/present/ future. Usually you will find, as we noted above, that the person occupies a very small slot of the continuum, where the attention is frozen or fixated on a small portion of the past. By expanding the past and the present, you automatically increase future potentialities and possibilities. By teaching the person how he is creating his subjective experience of time, you are teaching him that he can create a new experience of time. Here, time moves out of the realm of the absolute and into the private dominion of each individual.

Notice that I am again emphasizing process, not content. I am interested in *how* the person holds the past in the present, not in *what past contents* the person is holding. First and foremost I want to know: *Which Deep Trance Phenomena are you using to recreate your past in present time?* Secondarily I would want to know: What past *events* are you recreating in present time.

Once time distortion has been removed as a symptomatic trance, you can be taught to make use of it as resource. Say you are at a social gathering and you find yourself feeling bored. You realize that time is passing slowly, which is your cue to play with it. As you stand there holding your glass of wine, realize that there is no such thing as intrinsic drabness, or intrinsic discomfort, or intrinsic stupidity. All of those labels are assigned by each of us as consciously functioning beings. If things seem drab, then, and time drags along, realize that you are creating that particular experience. To begin altering it, ask yourself, Can I create a good time for myself here and now? Can I create an experience of time "flying by"? If the answer is no, you are still at the mercy of an autonomously functioning trance state. If the answer is yes, you are on your way to one of the most prized abilities in any spiritual discipline: the ability to be in charge of your subjective experience of time; the ability to exist outside of time as we know it.

As a therapist you can work with one event, one sensation, one feeling, one resource of any kind that was pleasurable but experienced as brief and insignificant and *lengthen it and expand it and bring it into present time*; there is a reciprocal shrinking of the unpleasurable portions of the continuum.

Erickson used time distortion to ratify trance, since it is a convincing way to "prove" to a person that something different has happened. He would also *suggest* an experience of time distortion and hypnotic dreaming to patients during the last few minutes of the session: days, weeks, years, a lifetime could go by in just those few minutes of clock time, during which the patient would learn whatever was needed. Since time distortion is an integral part of most symptomatic trance states, I will also make use of it in a similar manner. However, rather than working from the vantage point of "inducing" time distortion in a client, I assume that I am utilizing the client's ongoing unique distillation of time distortion *that is already present in the symptom structure*.

Treatment of Time Distortion

Three principles or axioms guide our work with the Deep Trance Phenomenon of time distortion:

(1) We create our experience of time in the body;
(2) We sustain our experience of time by putting it on "automatic";
(3) We can alter how we subjectively experience the sense of time we have created.

As I have said, time distortion is rarely a solitary trance. It is almost always part of a cluster of trance phenomena that coalesce to create the symptom. To identify if time distortion is part of your symptom, consider the following signposts:

(1) Feeling "frozen" or "stuck" around particular incidents in your life such as childhood trauma, divorce, death, separations, and so on. If you were divorced ten years ago, but the pain of it is still so vivid it seems like a recent experience, then you are making use of time distortion to hold the divorce process in present time and lengthen it way past its chronological reality.

(2) Chronic feelings of anxiety around the theme of "There is never enough time! I'm running out of time!" Here, time distortion has turned time itself into the enemy so that the person experiences it as hopelessly shortened.

(3) Chronic feelings of depression in which the time of each day seems to last forever. "Will this day never end" is the lament here, where time has become the enemy by taking forever!

Reversing Subjective Time

Step 1: Get in a comfortable position, lying down or sitting, close your eyes and recall an unpleasant experience in which you still feel stuck. Now *lengthen* it. Since you are used to lengthening unpleasant experiences, it makes sense to begin by taking control in a familiar direction. To ask you to shorten it first would put you in a position of resisting. This is basically an Ericksonian technique called "symptom prescription" in which the individual experiences control over an autonomous symptom by experiencing it *more*.

Step 2: Now recall a pleasant time in your life and *shorten* your experience of it. This continues the principle discussed above.

Step 3: Now reverse what you have been doing. While continuing to breathe deeply in a relaxed autohypnotic state, begin to lengthen your experience of the pleasant event and shorten your experience of the unpleasant one. Use all your imaginative powers to envision, for example, the early childhood trauma passing by quickly; and as it passes swiftly by, turn your imagination toward a leisurely experience of some pleasant event. Enjoy the pleasure from the event as it endures through days and weeks, all the way into the present moment.

To gain a sense of the degree to which we orchestrate our experience of time, see these two incidents—pleasant and un-pleasant—co-existing side by side. Now alternate your experience of them. Choose to lengthen the unpleasant while shortening the pleasant; choose to shorten the unpleasant while lengthening the pleasant. With focused attention notice how you gain increasing facility in alternating your own experience of time.

Recontextualizing Time

Step 1. After you have altered your own experience of your life events, you need to place those events back into the context of your unique existence. Let your unconscious mind produce an image for you that represents your entire life experience. For example:

(a) Imagine an ocean that contains your existence from beginning to end. Feel the expanse of your total life experience. Now take the newly lengthened and shortened incidents and place them in this unified ocean of existence. Step into the ocean and experience these incidents in relation to the new time-shifts you have created.

(b) If you prefer an image of outer space, create it as the context of your life experience, following the same instructions as above.

(c) Experience your time-shifted incidents being re-woven into a large tapestry.

(d) Use an image of a bouncing ball. See your entire life contained in the bouncing ball; the *down bounce* represents the shortened, unpleasant experience and the *up bounce* carries the lengthened, pleasant experience. Feel yourself bounce through life experiences staccato-like when they are unpleasant, long and languidly when they are pleasant.

(e) Visualize a sparkling, flowing mountain stream. Let the "leaves" or incidents of your life, which you have just experienced in a time-shifted modality, float into the stream of your existence. Let each "leaf" be carried along effortlessly and rhythmically, as your new time-oriented experiences are integrated into the context of present time.

Step 2. Once the newly recontextualized frozen event is placed in the context of your current life, ask the unconscious for an image or symbol of the self. Once the symbol is clear, visualize its appropriate position in the body and connect it to the recontextualized experience. This holds the new experience in the body as well as in a new ego-self.

Step 3. Create posthypnotic suggestions that make use of behavioral inevitabilities. Erickson and Rossi (1979) have described this technique of linking future reintegration with a behavioral inevitability such as eyes opening, sighing, stretching. For example, the suggestion might be given: "When and only when your conscious and unconscious mind agree to continue the work will your eyes open."

In the case of time distortion you can liken the lengthening or shortening of time to the inevitable experience of walking, whereby the right foot lengthens pleasant events and the left foot shortens unpleasant ones. Breathing can also be used: With each inhalation, pleasant events will naturally lengthen while unpleasant events shorten on the exhalation; or, perhaps pleasant events will lengthen on the exhalation while unpleasant events shorten on the inhalation.

Time is a major factor in trance phenomena. The *body* trance of time distortion freezes thoughts, feelings, emotions, and associations, thus locking them in a rigid body structure that reduces the flow of resources. Traumas, which are experienced in the body, must be addressed in the body in order to "un-freeze" the trance of time distortion that holds the past in present experience.

16

Hypnotic Dreaming

TO DAYDREAM is to go into trance. We have all experienced it hundreds of times. Daydreams and fantasy can be the stuff of creative genius, or they can shackle the dreamer to an unfulfilled life of empty yearnings. Some of us don't daydream enough; others daydream more than is helpful. Either way, for most of us, daydreams just come and go at will—*their* will, rather than our conscious will. We get what we need or want from them and then "wake up" and move on with daily life orientations.

For some, daydreaming or "hypnotic dreaming," another Deep Trance Phenomenon, has become a habitual response that functions so autonomously that it impedes adult living. The hypnotic dream is used to resist experiencing the present. Dreams of this nature are deeply layered in the age-regressed "child within" and become a prime impetus for entire adult lifestyles. The unaware adult incessantly and impotently daydreams about the future, not realizing that it is the "child within" who is creating and sustaining the over-idealized dream.

As with all other Deep Trance Phenomenon, hypnotic dreaming was created by the child to protect and maintain his integrity. In response to a stressful series of interpersonal interactions, the child dissociated from the outer environment as well as the inner self (who is afraid, in pain, unhappy, or whatever), went into an *intra*personal trance and created a dream or fantasy. Whenever a child is denied the essential ingredients for living, he will attempt to counter or neutralize the deprivation. This attempt may take the form of the creation of a dream character who gives the child the experience of security and wholeness he is seeking. I call this "externalization": needed experiences are dissociated and externalized or projected onto the outer world via imagination, dreaming, and fantasy.

Both the "child within" doing the dreaming and the dream itself remain time-frozen and dissociated. As the child grows older, the "dream" becomes increasingly inappropriate and unreal because it is a product of a young child's world, not the present adult world. The age-regressed "child within" can only interact as a child attempting to complete itself, not as an adult meeting his own needs. In addition, *intra*personal dreams lack *inter*personal feedback, which means that the dream continues without a reality check in the outer world.

For example, as a five-year-old girl is repeatedly spanked by her authoritarian father, she begins to defend herself from within by splitting off from the outer actions and by splitting off from the inner turmoil, and creating a dream in which she is rescued by a kind man who takes her to his royal kingdom where she is hailed as a princess. This dream brings her comfort—or, that is, it brings the dissociated "child within" comfort—and she begins to use it automatically, whenever she wants to feel better.

Twenty years later the child has become a woman who wants to have a serious relationship. But the "child within" continues to fantasize. Ironically, the dream itself draws her to abusive relationships because before she can be rescued and instated as a princess, she must first find herself in peril. Obviously, neither child nor adult recognizes the "dark" part of the dream that is the very genesis of the dream itself! Yet it is this dark (by *dark* I mean hidden—implied but not seen) part that actually winds up manifested.

The hypnotic dream is so woven into the fabric of her consciousness that she accepts it as a "given." For her, unconsciously the dream portrays what she has experienced to be the nature of reality, so she does not look for answers anywhere else. Furthermore, the "child within" is always operating, always ready to generate the rescue dream as salve, so there is no need to reach for something better.

Everyone has an inner child. Ideally, however, we are not dominated by it. We can become playful and silly at will, and then stop being playful and silly. We can cuddle and be cuddled, and also feel fine if we are not. The question to ask is, Am I automatically being thrown by this "child within" who... *has to have* an ice cream cone, who *has to be* held and cuddled, who *has to buy* a new dress? Or can I choose not to act? For the adult locked into hypnotic dreaming, there is no sense of choice—only of domination and compulsive need. Stated another way, the dreams and fantasies happen automatically, whether we want them or not.

The Feedback Loop Linking Dream and Context

Sometimes an adult's hypnotic dream will be manifested in his "real" outer life. This happens when the person has the talent and abilities to make the dream real. There is still an underlying process of dissociation and an ongoing trance of hypnotic dreaming sustaining the current success, but the person usually does not experience that as a problem.

For example, a young boy surrounded by quarreling parents who do not value education discovers that the one thing that gives him pleasure is books and the process of learning. Despite the hostile environment, which undermines rather than supports this passion, the child finds ways to learn as much as possible. Meanwhile, the Deep Trance Phenomenon of hypnotic dreaming is used to stave off the stress and unhappiness of a brutal father and an intimidated mother. The young boy is forever daydreaming of the time when he will have his own library, will write his own books, will give lectures and be heralded for his work. Even when his school performance is so poor he is put in the "dumb" class, his hypnotic dream sustains him.

If this child was not gifted in the directions he daydreamed, he would probably grow into an adult for whom hypnotic dreaming had become a symptomatic trance state. Being suitably gifted, however, the child begins to find ways to make the dream real.

Slowly, a "feedback loop" between the dream and his interpersonal world is formed. Over the years, the dream and the young man's lived life gain increasing correspondence. He may still be trying to prove that he is not "dumb"—and in that sense, he is still being dominated, to some degree, by his dream trance and by the unconscious hypnotic identity of "I'm dumb." But the fact that he *is* able to manifest the dream greatly diminishes its problem-generating powers.

More often, there is no feedback loop to support the dream. It floats in space, utterly disconnected from real-life experience. Los Angeles is like a magnet for hypnotic dreamers of the entertainment variety, who experience repeated rejections yet persevere with astonishing tenacity. Everyone is going to be an actress or an actor or a director or a screenwriter, but the feedback loop still has them working in restaurants, driving taxis, selling insurance. The closest they get to their dream is to take a course now and again.

I knew one embittered man who had read for parts in television and film hundreds of times over a ten-year period. He had not gotten one part, yet if you asked him what he did for a living, he would reply, "I'm an actor. I'm just doing real estate for the time-being." There is certainly nothing wrong with persevering to become an actor. The problem was that he denied having the job that netted his livelihood and paid his bills. He dissociated from his co-workers and felt unfulfilled at the workplace. Rather than dealing with this difficulty directly, he preferred to dream. He ignored the interpersonal loop of not receiving a part and felt unappreciated, unloved, and angry.

This man described a childhood dominated by *not having*. His parents were good people, there was no brutality in the house, but they lived in deprivation—which he loathed. To survive a chronic condition of impoverishment, he used hypnotic dreaming to give him a reason to live. As a child, he had developed the habit of dissociating from his undesirable surroundings and fantasizing glamorous ones. Interestingly, this very same mechanism is what kept him locked into failure in a profession for which he was entirely unsuited: Just as the child had dissociated from the feedback loop of *not having*, the adult dissociated from the feedback loop of *not getting*. Each time he was rejected for a part, he automatically flipped into his hypnotic dream. This is the point at which hypnotic dreaming, unsupported by a confirming feedback loop, becomes a symptomatic trance that impedes successful adult functioning.

Chronic adult "dreamers" rarely recognize that their fondest dreams are a trance state at the source of their problems. The hypnotic dreams that were created during childhood usually have been heavily reinforced with years of amassed "data" that supposedly supports the dream. Yet when the adult is confronted with the "fact" that the dream has never been manifested and is, in fact, quite cut off from real life, she will often react quite defensively, marshalling many "logical" explanations. In a way, the dreamer has a kind of co-dependent relationship with her dream: she can justify any flaw or failure with great facility! The dream represents an old ideal that was protective of the child's self, and the child does not want to give it up. In working with a client's hypnotic dream, efforts to integrate the other side of the dream (Prince Charming comes home late and drinks too much; rock stars are hounded by thousands of people; corporate presidents have no life of their own), feelings of grief, disillusionment, discontentment and confusion will arise. The dreamer does not want reality polluting her dream! The task for the therapist is to allow these emotional responses while not merging or becoming *entranced* by the client's emotional logic in support of the childhood dream. A brief example is discussed below, under Step 1 of "Treatment."

The Need for Hypnotic Dreaming

Hypnotic dreaming is a naturalistic trance phenomenon that can benefit us as long as we remain in charge. The question to be asked is, *Am I creating this dream or fantasy knowingly and purposefully, or is it happening "automatically"*? Healthy use of this Deep Trance Phenomenon lies in our ability to exercise creativity and choice. Choice means the ability to create or let go of our hypnotic dreams at will. For most people, their hypnotic dreams function on "automatic pilot" and are derivations of unfinished childhood issues. Restoring choice—*not* removing or suggesting away the dream itself—is the therapeutic task.

Clients may present with the opposite problem: a complete inability to dream or fantasize. If we recall a basic premise that a symptom is the *non*-utilization of unconsicous resources, then being unable to dream, daydream or fantasize also becomes a liability. I worked with a man who, as a result of being unable to daydream, lived in an overly linear, over-focused, over-identified state. He was criticized in his job for being "unimaginative" and warned that some improvement was expected.

He was extremely anxious when he arrived for his first session, explaining that he feared his job was "on the line" for something he had no control over. He firmly believed that he was incapable of daydreaming about anything and contended that "that kind of thinking that goes off into unreal, never-never lands" was foreign and even frightening to him. He rushed to explain that his father had been an alcoholic who terrorized their household of five. Being the oldest, he had assumed primary caretaking duties in an effort to give his mother some relief. To him, going off into a daydream meant abandoning everyone to the possibility of the father's rampages. His trance-response to the environmental and interpersonal stress was to remain hyper-alert at all times to be able to read the signs and take protective action at a moment's notice. This type of hypervigilant identity is often characteristic of homes where alcohol or drug abuse is present. An adult-child of an alcoholic often has to stay so *present* because to let go and fantasize could mean catastrophe.

Daydreaming is the wellspring of imagination and creativity. As an adult, this man needed to develop his ability to daydream, with *choice* added as the key ingredient. Both he and the obsessive daydreamer have the same therapeutic goal: to make use of this trance resource of hypnotic dreaming by choice rather than being barred from it or compelled into it.

I asked the client to sit comfortably and to breathe and look at me. Since he was used to being hyper-vigilant, it seemed easy for him to narrow his focus as I suggested. However, his familiar pattern was automatically broken by the added task of *breathing*. In his "unedited" hypervigilant state, he would hold his breath and tighten his muscles as he surveyed his surroundings. Now he was being asked to look *and* breathe at the same time. After a few minutes, his pupils began to dilate and his focus diffused to a distant set-point even as he continued to "breathe and look at me." Now I asked him to pick an image from nature that he liked and to see it in his "mind's eye." He picked a sea gull but said he couldn't see it. To depotentiate his negative ("I can't see it"), I assured him: "You're not supposed to be able to see anything but my face and the furniture yet. I don't know how long it will take to. . .see the sea gull inside your mind. Just continue to breathe and look at me."

A few minutes passed when he softly stated, "I can see it— faintly, behind a gray mist."

I immediately asked him to stop seeing the sea gull, and to see only those things that were "really" in his visual range. He looked puzzled but mumbled "okay."

"What do you see as you breathe and look at me?" I asked.

He responded by naming a few pieces of furniture.

Next I asked him to stop seeing the furniture and resume watching the sea gull as he breathed and looked at me.

He nodded absently and mumbled that the fog had cleared and there were actually three sea gulls now.

We continued this process for about 20 minutes, alternating between "real-world" sight and "inner-world" sight.

When he returned the following week he reported that he had felt "disoriented, but in a pleasant sort of way" throughout the week. As he spoke, I got an image of neurons being turned on in his brain for the first time. Nothing spectacular had happened—he hadn't suddenly wowed his boss with an ingenious solution to some corporate problem—but he nonetheless had the feeling that "something important was going on."

We continued to build these fantasy "highways" each session, adding on elements as he grew accustomed to the process. First he had to become accustomed to the experience/sensation of seeing with his "mind's eye" rather than with his physical eyes. (Visualization is not an automatic ability in people and can seem quite foreign and daunting. In my experience it has to be slipped in—with no special name or explanation and with no long descriptions of what it is.) Next he learned how to let the visualized image move and change a bit, but at a fairly uncomplicated level. Eventually, he was able to allow an entire "dream-story," as he called it, to unfold.

Meanwhile, back on the job his attitude changed subtly, which was enough improvement for his supervisor to give him some time and space. He began having an entirely new experience in which ideas "just floated" into his thoughts. He made no conscious connection between being able to see sea gulls inwardly and these

192 · Trances People Live

new floating thoughts. He was simply excited by it, said he felt much better, and quit therapy! Six months later he phoned to ask "if the sea gulls had anything to do with his new brain" and to tell me how pleased he was with his new ability.

Treatment of Hypnotic Dreaming

I. Returning Choice to Interruptive Hypnotic Dreaming

The overall therapeutic goal in working with hypnotic dreams that function automatically and disruptively is to re-unite the dream with its "other" more realistic side and join or integrate it with the "child within," the self, and the larger interpersonal context. I'll illustrate using a case example.

A man came to therapy with the complaint that he was always "in the red" and it was causing marital problems. He said he wasn't "*that* concerned" about his finances, except for occasional bouts of anxiety when the bills really accumulated. His wife, however, was "fed up" and gave him the ultimatum of therapy or divorce. It was she who was paying for the therapy.

He explained that he was "New Age" and that he didn't expect me to understand his thinking. I asked, "What is your thinking?" "I *imagine* money coming my way; I meditate and visualize all my bills being paid, and abundance surrounding us."

I said, "That's great, but do you *do anything* to manifest that belief in the outer, physical world?"

He said, "I spend money whenever I begin to worry about it— that manifests my belief in abundance."

"Oh, but do you look for employment? Are you adequately trained to work in the real world?"

"Not really."

"Would you like to be able to match your belief with your living circumstances?"

"Sure."

"Do you think it's possible you're leaving out an element or two in this cosmic approach—since you're not exactly abundant?"

"I suppose I must be. Do you know what it is?"

"I think it's *integration*, in a nutshell."

I have no quarrel with New Age teachings about the importance of beliefs, but what I do find amusing is how *disconnected* the teaching gets from the material, physical world. Hypnotic dreamers are prime candidates for this distortion, and this man was a classic example of the hypnotic-dreamer-turned-New-Age-disciple.

Because the dreamer is addicted to his childhood dream-state, which leaves the dream in a completely dissociated realm, the first goal in therapy, as mentioned above, is to reassociate or re-integrate four different planes of functioning: the "child within" who created hypnotic dreaming in the first place, the "opposite side" of the hypnotic dream itself, the self or ever-present core of the individual, and the outer world. *You do not want to simply discard the dream or even reframe it*—you want to integrate it or "ground" it (in Bioenergetic terms) into the body and the entire landscape of the person's psyche and social network.

In order for the intrapersonal trance of hypnotic dreaming to occur, the body must become ungrounded. This ungrounded feeling is a cornerstone of trance. Pioneer bodyworkers Wilhelm Reich and Alexander Lowen believe that the basic life energy must be discharged through the feet (as well as through orgasm). If this life energy does not have an avenue of discharge, it goes upward to the mind and creates thoughts, dreams, and fantasies. Reich believed that the less life energy was charged and discharged through the body, the less feelings could be experienced. Moreover, the greater the inhibition of energy discharge, the greater the tendency to mystify the world. The energy had to go somewhere, so it went "up," creating fantasies of gods and goddesses in extreme cases. This line of thinking also explains the practice of celibacy among the spiritual: the more celibate the life, the less discharge of life energy; and the less discharge, the more mystification.

Step 1: Integrate the "Opposite Side" of the Dream

I had a client whose dream was to be taken care of for the rest of her life by a wealthy millionaire. She firmly believed such a situation would solve all her problems of self-dislike and emotional instability. In trance I suggested to her that nobody is perfect, and chances are high that she would encounter the same round of trials and disappointments with her millionaire benefactor as any of us encounters with a spouse. Perhaps he will be a womanizer, staying out all night from time to time; perhaps he will be a workaholic who travels three-quarters of the month; perhaps he will expect her to cater to him hand and foot; perhaps he will behave quite dictatorially. The one sure bet is that no human being, including a millionaire, is going to be perfect; and the larger her dependency on him, the greater the chances of serious problems.

Needless to say, my client did not want me to talk along these lines. She recognized the hit of reality immediately and moved rapidly to resist it. She began by trying to name wealthy individuals from history who had also been "great human beings." When I suggested that she knew nothing of these men's personal lives, she admitted that was true and added, "but *surely* they were good to their wives!" Then she began to cry, which was her first real breakthrough. I had an image of her tears gently breaking up the unity of the dream.

A week later she came to therapy feeling more grounded in who she was, what she wanted, and most importantly, in the context that was available to her. Her feedback loop to the interpersonal world was leading her out of her intrapersonal fantasy.

Step 2: Create a Symbol

Typically the hypnotic dream is turned to in times of stress, so I begin by asking the person to duplicate the sensation of stress or pressure. In the case of the "New Age" client, I asked him to vividly recall the last time he sat in front of his bills and to describe his physical sensations "as you breathe and look at me." When he began to re-create the anxiety symptoms I said to him:

"I'd like to ask your unconscious mind for an image symbol of the YOU who is larger than the anxiety—perhaps you think in terms of 'higher self' or 'essential self' or 'soul' or 'spirit.' Whatever word you use, let your unconscious give you an image of it. Perhaps it is a mountain, or a river, or an animal—I don't know what it will be. But it will be interesting to see what image your unconscious gives you."

A good thirty seconds passed before he answered softly, "I see a tree."

Step 3: Place the Symbol inside the Body

Next I asked him to place the image of the symbol in some part of his body.

Another lapse of time and he responded almost inaudibly, "It goes in my heart."

Recall the discussion of expanding the context of the symptom to encompass the body, the self, and the social network in Chapter 6. Here, the symptom is not a localized pain or even a specific relationship. It is an intangible dream that is completely disconnected from the person's reality as a physical being. So I want to get him into his body, so to speak; I want to get him reconnected to the physical world. While the dream functions autonomously, there is no alignment between his Self, his body, and the outer world. The "spine" of this flow is out of kilter, so to speak.

Why don't I simply begin by giving him some practical suggestions for going out on a job interview? Because he is too dissociated to take that kind of action yet. He would just say, "Great, sure, yeah," and then go home and fantasize. First I want to integrate the dissociated trance by reconnecting it to an intrapersonal feedback loop in his body.

Step 4: Integrate Dream with the "Child Within"

Next I want the client to connect with the time-frozen "child within" who created the dream in all its varied forms, so I begin weaving back and forth between the image, the self, the child:

"As I look at the tree inside your heart I see a little child over there. . .a child climbing on a tree, in a tree house, looking down from the tree house. And there's Dad over there, but the child is way over here inside the tree. How safe it is to be in the tree, and what a nice game for a little child to play while in a tree house."

Step 5: Integrating the Social Network

To solidify the process of integration or grounding, I now extend the context of the therapeutic work to encompass a larger social network:

"And now, look, the child can see a tree inside of Dad. . .and there is that third-grade teacher, and she has a tree inside of her. . .And there is a tree inside of that little girl, Suzy. And as you sit there, isn't it nice to know that you can experience yourself in that tree inside your own body looking out and seeing another tree. And there are so many trees in the world, and so many woods, and the birds fly off and communicate to other trees and to other birds. And you can send birds from birds to birds, and how nice it is to know that you can house a whole family inside a bird's nest inside a tree."

Step 6: Integrate Image in Here-and-Now

To complete the process of re-integrating the trance of hypnotic dreaming, I suggest to the client that he visually place his resource in various locations in the room we are in, in his house, in his office, and so forth. The image of the self thus also becomes a symbol of this integration.

II. Facilitating Hypnotic Dreaming in Non-Dreamers
Step 1: First Visualizations

Have the client get into a comfortable position and ask her to "begin to imagine a pleasurable environment—perhaps the woods, the shoreline, a lake, a willow tree in a meadow." Explain to the client that this visualization is experienced by people in very unique ways: some "see" the scene quite vividly, while others might re-create it more kinesthetically by getting the sensations in the body. Still others who are more auditory in their sensory preference might hear the visualization more than see it.

Step 2: View from Above

Next have the client take a "look" from above so that he sees the outer edges, the boundaries, of the imagined scene. Placing a boundary around the new visualization helps to solidify it in form, making it more tangible, more discernible, and more manageable.

Step 3: View from Within

Now ask the client to step into the imagined scene and feel what it feels like to be part of the dream. Having the client merge with the characters in the dream—feel what it feels like to be them, hold their point of view, ideas, opinions, feelings, bodily sensations—makes the experience of the dream more grounded and real. Suggesting that they see the ocean, sky, land, or whatever, from behind the eyes of the dreamer gives the dream more substance and helps to dispel the disclaimer, "It was just a fantasy."

Step 4: Night Dreams

Suggest to the client that she ask her unconscious to allow her nighttime dreams to be remembered. As an exercise, write down the first conscious thought upon awakening. Do this for a period of several weeks and notice the accuracy of the insight from the dreams.

An advanced technique is to present the unconscious with a particular problem before falling asleep, and ask for a dream containing a solution.

Hypnotic dreaming is not "wrong." It is simply disruptive when it is allowed to function autonomously because the individual loses connection to his own body, to his deeper self, and to his interpersonal context. It is by re-establishing these interconnecting pathways that the individual can once again feel "in charge" of the automatic fantasizing rather than feeling like a victim of his own created trance phenomenon.

17

Sensory Distortion

SENSORY DISTORTION is a physical experience in which sensations are either amplified and overly sensitized or dulled and desensitized. The distortion is that the sensation, rather than being experienced in its "pure form," is somehow altered to protect the individual. In cases of abuse, for example, numbness will be used to provide the person with the feeling that "it never happened" or that the physical pain "didn't bother me." The actual sensory experience of the abusive event—the pain, injury, and physical assault on the child's body—is thus physiologically altered through a protective Deep Trance. The resulting trance of sensory distortion is put on automatic, to be called upon whenever the child is threatened or harmed.

For the adult, the habitual use of sensory distortion will interfere with intimate relationships, cause psychosomatic symptoms, sexual dysfunctioning, and make environmental stimuli needlessly stressful. The therapeutic goal in working with sensory distortion as a Deep Trance Phenomenon is to dissolve the trance by differentiating it.

This approach differs somewhat from Erickson's work, in that Erickson was more inclined to reframe, restructure, and/or utilize the client's sensory experience. The sensations involved in pain, for example, could be depotentiated by the more pleasant experiences of therapeutic trance and then more fully disarmed by creative reframing. The pain is reframed as a signal (Rossi, 1986) or solution (Gilligan, 1987), or restructured as an annoying itch, for example.

Typically, however, the experience of sensory distortion has not been recognized or worked with as a Deep Trance Phenomenon per se. Gilligan has noted the sensory alterations that characterize symptomatic trances, but his approach, like Erickson's, is to reframe and/or utilize the distortion. For example, in working with a woman who developed complete tunnel vision whenever her husband interacted with other women, Gilligan describes an approach in which "the jealous client was taught to hypnotically utilize tunnel vision in a variety of self-valuing ways, including focusing on her husband in a fashion that elicited a variety of secure and pleasurable feelings" (p. 53).

I prefer to "clean the slate," so to speak, and simply remove the trance from its habitual reign rather than allowing it to remain, even if reframed. A reframed trance is still a trance —which means it is an unnecessary "lens" that shrinks and narrows the person's perspective. Dissolving a Deep Trance Phenomenon from its habitual reign does not mean exiling it: the person still can choose to make use of this particular trance in a situation of need but is not tied to it by autonomous functioning. A person attempting to lose weight, for example, could use this trance selectively to alter the sensations of hunger. A performer could use it to lessen or dissipate the sensations of "stage fright."

In clinical work I have encountered three different types of sensory distortion:

(1) *psychophysiological sensory distortion* in which unwanted sensations are numbed, dulled, or overly intensified;

(2) *hyper- or hypo-sensory distortion* in which environmental stimuli are amplified or obliterated;

(3) *pain sensory distortion* in which only the afflicted portion of the body is perceived.

Psychophysiological Sensory Distortion

A man weighing 300 pounds came to me for the problem of obesity. I asked him to "breathe and look at me," and he began to "space out," to dissociate, and to experience his body as a "rock" or "stone" (sensory distortion). There was no sense of movement in this sensation; in general, he was unable to perceive sensations throughout his body, or, when they arose, he dulled them with food.

I began by suggesting that he "feel a sensation and then experience a space, feel another sensation and then a short space, feel another sensation and a long space." In this way he could "dip his toe" into the world of sensation with plenty of safe spaces in-between. In essence, he had developed a total body anesthesia as a defense against feeling. I wanted to introduce him slowly to this unfamiliar world.

Eventually, the undifferentiated mass that was his body began to throb and pulsate. As I continued, he began to take charge unconsciously of the "rock dead" feeling of protection by lengthening or shortening the gaps between sensations, as he preferred. Lengthening the gap slowed or lessened the sensations; shortening the gap heightened the sensations. As a result of this process, the client rapidly developed greater feeling for his body; he could no longer *not feel* his body. On his own, he began walking and watching his diet, and over a long period of time, continued to lose weight slowly.

Premature ejaculation in men is an example of psychophysiological sensory distortion in which sensations are overly intensified and localized—in this case, at the tip of the penis. Changing the pace and the rhythm of the sensations, together with spreading them throughout the body, serves a dual purpose of overcoming the premature ejaculation and enhancing the person's overall sexual experience far beyond what it was to begin with.

Begin by slowing down the sensations at the tip of the penis, and then suggest a greater gap between the sensations. In premature ejaculation the penis is dissociated from the rest of the body, as all of the person's attention centers on it. Once you begin to get gaps between the sensations, you get a more dispersed experience of throbbing and an increased ability to sustain the pulsations without coming to a premature orgasm.

This particular technique can be used by anyone who wants to enhance his or her experience of the self during sexuality. It is a simplification of the Eastern method of Tantric sex, in which sensations typically experienced in localized areas (genitals, mouth, breasts, etc.) are extended throughout the entire body. Sexual sensations are then felt in elbows, ankles, toes, forearms, and so forth. This kind of sexual experience de-emphasizes orgasm and focuses on an equal distribution of sexual energy throughout the body. When this practice is continued, the utilized energy created through sexual contact allows successive plateaus to be reached in which ever deeper experiences of the self are created.

It is interesting to note that the Tantric (Eastern) approach to sex and the Reichian (Western) approach to sex vary quite markedly in this regard. In his research on sex and orgasm, Wilhem Reich isolated the orgastic cycle as *tension—charge—discharge—relaxation*. Success in Reichian Therapy was achieved when a person could reach orgastic potency.

In Tantric sex, by contrast, the sexual charge is *not* discharged. The cycle in Tantric sex would be comprised of: *tension—charge— turning attention toward the sensations and seeing them as made of energy or consciousness—moving to another level of awareness.* The Tantric "plateaus" would continue to move "up" by utilizing the sensations and allowing them to spread throughout the body and into higher states of understanding *(consciousness)*. The *Vijñana bhairava* states, in essence, that if at the moment of orgasm you were to become introverted, you would experience divine consciousness. The bases of these differing approaches to working with sexual sensation will be elaborated in my forthcoming book, *Quantum Consciousness: The Discovery and Birth of Quantum Psychology: The Physics of Consciousness.*

Hyper- or Hypo-sensory Distortion

A woman came to me complaining of her problem in groups. She was hypersensitive to "everyone's energy" and experienced rapid sensations in her heart and chest. I asked her to re-create these sensations as she breathed and looked at me. Once she had described the experience, I suggested that she begin to *slow down the sensations so that she would experience less sensation.* Changing the pace at which she was accustomed to experiencing her hypersensitivity was a way of altering her subjective experience. An additional suggestion was made that "you do not need to feel the feelings you don't need, and you can feel only the ones that are appropriate to the

situation, and that your unconscious can decide which is which."
This subtle suggestion for negative kinesthetic hallucinations gave
her a tremendous sense of relief—she didn't *have to* feel it all.

Pain Sensory Distortion

Sensory distortion almost inevitably emerges in direct relationship to the experience of physical pain. The Deep Trance
Phenomenon shrinks the focus of one's attention to only the pained
area of the body. The entire remaining "field" of the body thus
becomes a non-utilized resource in which sensory flow is either
blunted or ignored.

Classic Hypnotic Anesthesia. The classic hypnotic approach in
working with pain is to induce hypnotic anesthesia or analgesia.
Kay Thompson, D.D.S., a student of Erickson, developed the
method of asking the patient to draw a mental circle around the
painful area and then to see the area as if it were transparent. The
patient could gaze upon the internal workings of the tissue—the
wiring of the nerves, in particular—and imagine those nerves
carrying the painful sensations all the way to the brain. Through
suggestion, the brain is likened to a computer room or telephone
switch board where all the wiring in the body connects. Then, with
permission from the patient's unconscious, the patient is given
suggestions to disconnect the wires that are connected to the painful
areas.

Ericksonian Approaches. Erickson and Rossi (1979) have
noted how difficult it is to induce true anesthesia, recommending
instead "the building of psychological and emotional situations that
are contradictory to the experience of pain and which serve to
establish an anesthetic reaction to be continued by posthypnotic
suggestion" (p. 98). Erickson was a self-taught master of pain
control and created many effective techniques such as the utilization of amnesia and/or dissociation, the replacement or substitution
of sensations, displacement of the pain, reinterpretation of it, use of
time distortion to alter the subjective experience of it, and so forth.

I have found two of these particularly helpful: the method of
differentiating the pain via description and division, and working
with the subjective experience of time in relationship to pain. In the

first method the pain, which is typically experienced as a block of undifferentiated experience, is divided and depotentiated via a series of questions. Say the patient initially describes his pain as "sharp." Ask, "Which part of the pained area is the sharpest? The left or the right? Which part of the pain area is the most interesting? Which part the most unusual?" This differentiation automatically changes the patient's subjective experience of the pain.

Another key, as Erickson pointed out, is to explain to the patient that pain is experienced in three temporal parts: (1) as past remembered pain, (2) as pain in the present moment, (3) and future imagined pain in which there are consequences as the pain continues (Erickson & Rossi, 1979). By focusing the patient on only that portion of the experience of pain that exists in the present—by excluding past remembered and future imagined pain—much of the present pain can be diminished.

I have found the use of head movements to be very helpful in communicating these different temporal relationships to pain. I emphasize my suggestions regarding past remembered pain by looking over the patient's left shoulder; the present is underscored by direct eye contact; and the future is reinforced by a head movement toward the right shoulder. By moving in conjunction with specific temporal suggestions, you are "marking out" for the unconscious mind its *lack of connection* to past and future pain.

Another effective Ericksonian tool for pain control is the use of multiple meanings, puns, jokes, metaphor, and reassociations that give the pain new, more tolerable meaning. Much is written on the subject, both by Erickson as well as his students, so there is no need to discuss it at length. The one point to remember is that there is no formula to create multiple meanings—and many therapists may feel no resonance with the technique whatsoever. It is simply one more tool. One brief example of how I have applied multiple meanings in working with pain control is that of a woman complaining of pain during her menstrual period. The pain centered in the area of her *colon* and would cause her to double-over with discomfort—a reaction that was further intensified by overwork.

My first suggestion to her was: "Do you know what a *period* is? A period is a time to pause before you go on, and if you *double* one period on top of another, you get a colon (:)—another kind of pause." This was the beginning entry point for changing her attitudes toward her period.

A psychologist friend of mine provided her own creative reassociations for her pain. She was scheduled to undergo a DNC. Prior to receiving this treatment, she identified several old emotional issues in her life and symbolically placed them into her uterus. Receiving only local anesthesia, she imagined the procedure to be cleaning out her "old stuff" and reported a feeling of euphoria during the process. She had created new meanings for the surgical experience and remained comfortably dissociated as she watched from her new perspective.

Symbols. I have developed a simple technique of evoking symbols to help in pain control. I ask the client to ask his unconscious for a symbol (such as a mountain, river, tiger, flower, pyramid, etc.) that will help reduce the pain, and then I offer the suggestion that the symbol be placed into the painful area of the body. As mentioned earlier, I myself was scheduled for a dreaded tooth extraction, so I created the symbol of Adolf Hitler having the tooth extracted instead! It was painless for me to watch Hitler having his tooth extracted.

Actually, the full story of my experience makes another important point, which is the need to make an agreement with your unconscious that you will deal with the pain in appropriate ways as soon as you can. In the meantime, you are asking it for anesthetic intervention. I had awakened in the middle of the night with severe tooth pain and had immediately induced my own hypnotic anesthesia. It was so effective that I "forgot" to make a dental appointment the next day. Halfway through the middle of the third day, my tooth and entire lower jaw erupted in excruciating pain and I had to receive emergency dental treatment. The moral is: You can learn to decrease and control the experience of pain, but you must not take advantage of the ability by withholding necessary medical or dental treatment. My unconscious would not allow me to use anesthesia after this experience, and I was stuck with massive dental work for months after that.

In working with the complaint of pain, I still tend to look for symptomatic clusters of Deep Trance Phenomena to see how the person is creating his or her unique experience of pain and then work with those trances.

For example, a woman came for therapy with the complaint of

chronic neck pain. I asked her to "breathe and look at me" while she described the sensations. She sat silent for several minutes and then spoke softly and like a little girl.

"The world is going to collapse," she said.

I told her to "continue to breathe and look at me" while she described the sensations in her neck. She paused again and then began speaking in her adult voice saying, "It hurts all over. . .I can't stand it. . .I hate it. . .I hate myself in pain. . . ." And so on.

What she was giving me was not so much a description of the sensations of pain in her neck as a reiteration of the posthypnotic suggestions she gave herself in response to the pain. I took a three-pronged approach. Since the suggestions seemed to work over her need to describe the pain, I began to differentiate the sensations of pain for her, while also shifting her own posthypnotic suggestions.

I asked, "Where do the sensations feel sharper? Where do the sensations feel duller? Where are the sensations burning? Where are they cool? Where are the sensations more concentrated? Dispersed?" (I repeatedly used the word *sensation* rather than *pain* to help shift her focus.) Meanwhile, I turned her self-induced posthypnotic suggestions into questions:

"I hate it?"

"I can't stand it?"

Then I split her suggestion "It hurts. . .all over," using a vocal emphasis that implied the hurt was *all over*, as in finished. This was followed immediately by a deluge of multiple meanings to create new associational networks as pathways to her unconscious: "I hate it. . .I ate it. . .I mate it. . .I rate it. . .I date it. . .I skate it. . . ."

Finally, I dispersed the pain throughout her body: "Just as sensations can move from your right index finger to your elbow, to your shoulder, to your head, you can let me know when the sensations in your neck begin to move into your shoulders, not to mention down your arms and hands." Eventually, the sensations of pain in her neck are equally distributed all over her body, thus relieving the neck area.

But who wants pain throughout the body? Localized pain sensations occur when, in Gestalt terms, the figure (in this case, the neck) is separated from the ground (the rest of the body). By suggesting movement of the sensations, I am reconnecting the figure (neck) to the ground (body) and simultaneously *expanding the focus of attention.* The Deep Trance Phenomenon is thus interrupted and thoroughly differentiated—which automatically dissipates the sensations of pain. Paradoxically, dispersing the localized pain throughout the entire "field" causes it to disappear altogether. To reiterate two axioms:

> *The greater the variability introduced into any symptom structure, the less fixed its outcome.* More simply put: *The more you add, differentiate, or vary a symptom, the less in tact it remains.*

> *There can be no Deep Trance Phenomena, and hence no symptom, without a shrinking of the focus of attention.*

A brief example continues to illustrate our two axioms. A client complained that he had experienced only emotional pain in his life, and that the pain was physically focused in his stomach. I suggested that "he might experience a desirable sensation in his hand or foot and a painful sensation in another part of his body." His head nodded slowly as I gave these suggestions. After the pleasant and unpleasant sensations were distributed equally, I suggested that he notice the sensations *moving* and *blending*. (Lack of movement was a chief characteristic of his chronic stomach pain, so introducing the experience of sensory movement was important.)

"And as the sensations move, they can...mingle...tingle...singling out a new experience."

Using this interspersal approach in which opposite sensations were offered allowed the client to expand his focus of attention and experience himself in an entirely different way. The integration of pleasant and unpleasant experiences yielded a third unique experience of sensation that had not been previously available. An excerpt of one trance period is as follows:

"I notice that you have a stomach, and that there is a stomach ache, and that's extremely painful. But you do have a hand and you can hold that hand, and it's nice to know that you can get a handle, and it's a handy way to hold something, as a pen in hand, or you can take a pen in hand and make a note. And there is sensation, a particular sensation around the pen, and a feeling—I don't know exactly if you'd call it certainty or security or maybe just confidence in knowing that you can hold that particular pen, write the way you're holding it as you breathe and look at me. Now you've got something in your stomach, a different sensation, not so pleasant, where am I going, what am I doing, where am I and who am I in my life. But I can feel the certainty in my hand, I can feel the certainty in my hand."

Treatment of Sensory Distortion

In addition to the approaches described for pain control, a number of simple exercises can be used as entry points to undifferentiated trances of sensory distortion. You can:

(1) speed up or slow down the sensations;

(2) expand and contract the gaps or spaces between individual sensations;

(3) ask your unconscious to select and allow you to feel only those sensations that are appropriate to your needs and situation;

(4) distribute the sensations equally throughout the body;

(5) create a pleasant sensation in one part of your body and a mildly unpleasant sensation in another part; mix and mingle the two until a third, entirely new sensation emerges.

As has been stressed throughout the text, sensations themselves are not only created by us, but their meaning and significance are also determined by us as the creators. Once we understand the subjective nature of sensations—their effects on us and our ability to change those effects—their "hold" and autonomy is diminished or removed entirely.

18

Differentiating and Reassociating the Trigger

I N DISCUSSING the various Deep Trance Phenomena, I have spoken frequently about the technique of differentiating the symptomatic trance state. In this chapter we are going to explore how a Deep Trance Phenomenon is activated by what I call the "trigger" mechanism, and then how to depotentiate it via differentiation and reassociation. By working with *both* the trigger and the resulting Deep Trance Phenomenon, you are "clearing the slate"— both internally, by removing the self-to-self symptomatic trance, and externally, by disassembling the self-to-other trance of the trigger. Another way of saying this is to say that you are integrating the *intra*personal trance (self-to-self) with its larger context or *inter*personal trance (self-to-other-environment).

This concept of working with both levels of trances helps to bridge the classic dichotomy of the intrapersonal and the systemic that has characterized the field of therapy since its origins. Psychotherapies tend to place themselves in either/or camp: they either focus *intra*personally, helping the individual gain insight into the interior functionings of his/or private psyche, or they contend that systems and larger contexts (families rather than individuals) are the only valid arena for work.

In the model I am proposing, the intrapersonal and interpersonal co-exist peaceably and with equal validity. Both aspects of reality—the inner and the outer—are inherent in symptom structures and beautifully mirror one another. One can always lead to the other—the intrapersonal can point you toward its interpersonal counterpart, or the reverse—but excluding either leads to incomplete approaches.

I define a *trigger* as an exterior stimulus that activates or catalyzes the internal response of a symptomatic Deep Trance Phenomenon(a). Consider, for example, the case of a woman who was molested as a little girl. In response to the assault, the little girl creates a protective trance of one kind or another, so the *trigger for this trance* is, initially at least, the man who molested her. Fear surrounds this trigger and she resists experiencing it even as it is internalized. Perhaps denial or amnesia are produced to help her tolerate the intolerable fact that the man who molested her was her uncle or her father or her older brother. The continual resistance to recognizing the trigger (the molester) is what holds it in her psyche for decades; she literally takes it with her through the years and events of her life, though in veiled form. The cloud of amnesia protecting her from specific identification causes her to project her fear outward, so that it lands in a generalized and inexplicable manner on men as a category. In high school she is terrified of being asked to dance but doesn't know why; she turns down requests for dates or goes on them but is miserably tense; by college she has struck out to liberate herself through sexual promiscuity but still finds no release from her fear; by adulthood she has a history of failed relationships and major depressive periods. This long history of difficulty is the result of the dynamic interaction of *intra*personal and *inter*personal processes that function like a cybernetic feedback loop. To restate this circular process:

(1) The trigger is internalized during the trauma;
(2) The trigger is resisted because it is painful or threatening;
(3) This resistance keeps the trigger "alive" internally;
(4) The resisted trigger is projected outward and generalized.

Reassociating the Trigger

When I first listen to clients describe their situations, each word they use tells me how they create their internal experience. By listening to the words they use to create their problems or symptoms, I can begin to alter the "groove" of their symptom-record by giving them new meanings and associations. Gradually, a different "tune" or inner state emerges as the meanings that form the foundation of the symptom structure are altered. In time, new associations create new outcomes, new behaviors, new internal realities.

Trust your own unconscious. If you allow yourself to "let go" into the interaction between yourself and your client, you will naturally enter a trance state in which associations pop up without conscious effort. Express these associations, offer them to the client; the more material you make available, the greater the flow of information between the two of you. Some of your associations will be on target, many will be off, but what counts is your own openness to the flow from your unconscious. If you begin to censor this internal process, you will find yourself feeling increasingly "stuck"; you have literally interrupted the outward flow of motion from your own psyche.

Rossi used the metaphor of lock and key to describe the probing associational process Erickson would go through in his hunt for the on-target therapeutic associations. He would try out dozens of metaphors, puns, jokes, and reassociations, knowing full well that only a small percentage stood a chance of functioning as the *key* to *unlock* the person's internal symptom structure. This is the point at which we are again reminded that *there is no formula for doing hypnotherapeutic work*. No matter how many training seminars, conferences, and workshops we attend, we cannot learn to do hypnosis in a step-by-step fashion because our unconscious perceptions do not flow in such a linear fashion. Certainly any study of Erickson's methods of working consistently reveal the frustrating (from a teaching point of view) fact that his interventions, responses, remarks, and behavior were never predictable. This was because he followed the circuitous, roaming, expansive, exploratory pathways of his own unconscious perceptions and processes *as they constellated in response to each unique individual.*

In my own experiences as a therapist I have maintained what might be viewed as a self-centered motive: I am there for my own growth. How can I make sure I grow? I set my own challenge of being able to totally "let go"—to merge simultaneously with the client and with myself—to let go of any resistance and any role-playing. Furthermore, I note places within myself where I feel "stuck" to a point of view or an automatic reaction. This is later used for my own personal work. I believe that my task is to let go of any preconceived outcomes or agendas. By doing this, it seems to free up the client's frozen point of view. If I don't know what to do in a session, I don't pretend that I do know, and I don't resist the experience of *not knowing*. I include myself in the trance process and I state where I am "at." I might say to the client:

"I don't know exactly what I'm doing, and I don't know exactly what to say, but I do know that my arms are crossed and I do know that my ankles have crossed one foot over the other. And I do know that I can take a lot of steps, and a lot of times things cross over, and my voice can cross over, and my words can cross over, with meaning."

Obviously, the above reflects my own particular needs and preferences. Each therapist must find his or her own way of grappling with the challenge of following their own unconscious associations, and sometimes of not knowing what to do.

Erickson's hypnotherapeutic work, which focused on creating new associational networks that "created a system of mutual support and momentum for initiating and carrying out a therapeutic pattern of responses," certainly forms the foundation of the approaches described in this chapter. However, there is an important difference in therapeutic goals: I am specifically focusing on a process that is intended to go beyond a trigger mechanism for a *symptomatic trance*, whereas Erickson's use of associational networks was more intended to create a state of *therapeutic trance*.

Case Example

A man came to see me in regard to relationship problems. He was "positive" that the woman he had been involved with for several years was going to break up with him. He had been married for 15 years, when his wife left him for another man. For seven years after his divorce, he allowed himself to engage in only one-night stands. Then he met this special woman and become emotionally involved. For the past two years, they had been living together "on and off," with marriage discussed as a probable but uncertain future.

Meanwhile, he had begun to obsess that "I'm afraid she is going to leave me." I worked with them both as a couple and individually, so I knew what position the woman held in the relationship, and I knew that his obsession was not based in any outer reality. He had a history of women leaving him, and he used that history to forecast his future, with the help of a little trance state called pseudo-orientation in time. What I wanted to know as the therapist was how this man was creating the *intra*personal experience called "She is going to leave me" in the *inter*personal context and interaction with his partner. He is creating his experience intrapersonally, self-to-self, but it is occurring in an interpersonal, self-to-other context.

I began by asking him, "What triggers this response inside you?" I then explained what I meant by using a personal example. What follows is a partial transcription of the session.

> *Therapist*: If I am driving down the street and I see a police car in front of me, I tighten my muscles and barely breathe. The policemen is the *trigger* for my body response of anxiety, and even though nothing has happened yet, I respond as if it had. So, what I'm asking is, what is your trigger in relation to Mary? What behavior in particular sets you off into the state of "She is going to leave me"?
>
> *Client*: Well, she hugs me. When we greet each other after coming home from work, she goes like this [*demonstrating*]—she taps me on the back or puts an arm around me. I can tell that it's becoming more of a friendship than a love relationship. I can sense it.
>
> *Therapist*: So her hand and the way she touches you triggers your response?
>
> *Client*: Yes.
>
> *Therapist*: You interpret her touch to be friendly rather than sexual?
>
> *Client*: Yes.
>
> *Therapist*: [*Beginning to differentiate the trigger*] Which finger feels most friendly?

Client: The middle finger.
Therapist: Which finger is the most sexual?
Client: The index finger.
Therapist: Which finger is the most affectionate?
Client: The ring finger.
Therapist: Which finger is the most interesting?
Client: The pinkie.
Therapist: And what about the thumb?
Client: It doesn't have any real purpose. It's just there to pick things up.
Therapist: So when she wants to pick up on you, you can feel it in the thumb? [*A suggested reassociation*]
Client: Well, I guess so.
Therapist: I don't have to tell you that in America, this gesture means one thing [*waving goodbye*], while this gesture [*motioning hand toward body, "come here"*] means something else. In India, waving goodbye actually means hello, and this gesture [*using hand and finger movements*] means, "I want to go to the bathroom." In New York, this gesture [*middle finger extended*] means "Fuck off," and this one [*thumb up*] means, "Give me a ride."

Throughout this passage I am attempting to differentiate the client's trigger—the particular touch of his partner's hand—into many different parts with many different meanings. I am creating experiential options as to what her hand means. I did not take away the client's reality that her touch meant "friends only," but I narrowed it down to only one finger, with other fingers meaning other things. Whenever a trigger is activated, it means that the person is shrinking his focus of attention down to one or two details and not seeing the entire person or event. In essence, even to perceive the trigger, the person has to go into trance. As the therapist, I want to expand the focus of attention and then differentiate (depotentiate) the trigger.

In another case, I worked with a man who had a history of drug abuse and who describe himself as unworthy: "Whenever I meet somebody, I always feel like they are going to reject me. I feel I am less then them, that I am unworthy."

He proceeded to describe an event that had occurred just prior to the session. He had gone to the store to buy some items. After selecting the items he walked toward to check-out counter, saw the clerk, and immediately felt agitated and inferior. I wanted to know exactly what triggered this response.

> *Therapist*: Was it the man's posture? His height? His coloring? Was it the way he held his mouth? The shape of his neck? The look in his eyes?
> *Client*: His eyes.
> *Therapist*: His left eye or his right eye?
> *Client*: His left eye.
> *Therapist*: Which part?
> *Client*: The part that wrinkles below the eye.
> *Therapist*: Which part of this man's face is the most accepting? Which part is saying, "Go away? You are not worth anything." Which part is saying, "Hi. How are you doing today?"

In this methodical manner I went through each part of the face and asked about meanings. The client was focusing on about 1/25th of what was present in this man's expression and giving it a particular meaning. Then, because I knew from his history that his alcoholic father was the initial trigger, I went through the same process to differentiate the trigger of his father's face. The more variations on any problematic experience that you can provide, the more choices you are simultaneously offering. Now when this client looks at a man's face and feels that internal response of "I'm going to be rejected," he immediately expands his focus systematically: he glances at the cheeks and gets a message of, "I'm worthy"; he glances at the mouth which says, "I care about you"; or at the forehead that says, "I'm having a hard day."

After this thorough process of differentiation, I ended the session by metaphorically reassociating the trigger, by creating an entirely new associational network, briefly as follows:

"If you were to divide the face like the face of the earth is divided, you would see these little lines, faces of the earth, latitude, longitude, and there are marks down the middle. You can look at the South Pole; you can look at a globe—round, like a face or a head, and so many different types of weather—cold, warm, water spots, snow spots, desert spots."

The basic rule is: *Differentiate and reassociate.*

Treatment of the Trigger

(1) Create new associations to the trigger stimulus that activate different (non-symptomatic) responses, as illustrated throughout this chapter.

(2) Expand the focus of attention to encompass the larger *context*. As illustrated in the case examples, the trigger is usually an isolated portion of a much larger "field." By allowing the perception of the entire field, latent resources emerge in the form of new perceptions, new feelings, new attitudes.

(3) Join each new association to what Erickson and Rossi (Erickson, Rossi, & Rossi, 1976; Erickson & Rossi, 1979) termed a "behavioral inevitability," thus creating new outcomes. For example, you might give the following posthypnotic suggestion:

"I don't know when you'll experience that sense of comfort. It might be when you see the sun, feel a breeze on your face, see the clouds, look in a mirror. I just don't know when you'll experience that feeling, but it will be interesting to notice *when you continue* to notice the whole face or the whole situation."

The phenomenon of the trigger is an excellent example of one of my guiding axioms:

The more the attention is narrowed and decreased, the more the person's choices and resources are narrowed and decreased.

This axiom appears to contradict a major thrust of Erickson's work, which was to purposely narrow the client's attention in therapeutic trance as a means of evoking unconscious resources. These two approaches are not really contradictory so much as based on differing assumptions. Because I view the symptom as a trance state and assume the person's attention is already in that narrowed state, I work to expand the focus of attention out of trance, whereby resources automatically emerge. Erickson viewed the trance state as therapeutic—which I agree, it can be—and therefore used it as his springboard into creating an expanded experience for the client. Either way—Erickson's therapeutic trance state or my no-trance state—the client's focus of attention is expanded.

19

The Formation Of Hypnotic Identities

I N PSYCHOLOGY it is common to talk about how one's sense of self is formed—one's *identity*. What is uncommon is the realization that many of the identities people casually own as being representative of who they are, are actually *trance identities*.

Like all Deep Trance Phenomena, a trance identity is created by the child as a means of self-preservation and to handle various problems and traumas. This identity is comprised of the child's assumptions and beliefs about his interactions with his parents: "*This* is how I should be...*That* is how I should not be...This is who I am." Psychologically speaking, the child fuses with the parents and creates an identity that reacts, thinks, sees, and hears either *like* the fused parent or *in resistance to* the fused parent. As adults, these identities remain on "automatic pop-up" and continue to function, seemingly autonomously, in relation to the early family context.

A simplistic example of this fusion process is the example of the young child viewing his alcoholic father being confronted by his enabling mother. The child "takes a picture" of the content and texture of these interactions, and like computer software, retains the

217

information within his developing consciousness. As an adult in search of an intimate relationship, the internal picture and content of the parents' relationship pop up, and the person proceeds to match his new partner with the internal "software."

As discussed in Chapter 14, the Deep Trance Phenomenon of confusion is the pivotal bridging mechanism in the creation of hypnotic identities. To briefly reiterate: Confusion is the transitional state in which a person shifts out of his real self and into the creation of defensive or compensatory identities. In order to "get clear," the person resists his initial trance of confusion by creating a part of himself—an identity—whose goal is to "get clear." Interestingly, I have found that other Deep Trance Phenomena do not seem to spawn hypnotic identities, although they can keep the identity functioning. For example, amnesia is definitely working as denial in the incest survivor who, during the molest, experienced confusion and created an identity of "It-never-happened." But *confusion* seems to be the primary "trance substance" fueling this unique psychological process of identity formation.

Roles and self-images are also part of the fabric of hypnotic identities that are created in the transition space of confusion (even though it may not seem so in the present): "I'm a writer," "I am a mother," "I'm an attorney," "I am a loser," "I'm a therapist," "I'm a stepfather," "I'm an athlete." Some identifications are much stronger than others, and these create what we label to be problems.

To be in a trance identity means that we have fused or become one with that experience, just as the child originally fused with the parent. Whether that identity is "I am a loser" or "I am a competent editor," in both cases one's experience of self is being *narrowed down*. There is a self behind the trance identity that is much "larger." If I can pick up and put down the trance identity I call "Stephen," then I am free of it. But if I pick it up and *can't* put it down, then I think that is all I am, and I shrink my focus of attention by limiting myself to that narrow conception.

We can talk about four different categories of trance identities: *role identities, professional identities, self-image identities,* and their corollary offspring: *oppositional identities.*

Role identities include all our social and familial functions: mother, father, wife, husband, stepmother, stepfather, community leader, environmental activist. It is easiest to see the identification with role identities in families—usually with the parents—when they have little or no sense of themselves as separate from the activities, accomplishments, problems, and dreams of their children.

I was at a party once where two women, each the mother of three grown children, got into a conversation about Mother's Day. Their interaction was a vivid depiction of the continuum of trance role identities. Norma began the conversation by making a lighthearted reference to her disdain for Mother's Day. She did not like the heavy role identification linked with the day and did not want to be "honored" in that way one bit. Her mothering identity was clearly something she could pick up and put down. Louise, by contrast, jumped in with an impassioned objection, heatedly defending her right to be honored as a mother. She liked the identification, felt threatened by having it taken away from her, and definitely did not want to put it down.

Professional identities span the gamut from plumber to professor, from dancer to electrician, from editor to gardener. We all have work/career identities of one sort or another. The aspect to monitor is the degree of identification we feel—the degree to which we can or cannot "pick it up and put it down." If you can't "put down" your worker identity, it means that your sense of selfhood and well-being are limited to your work abilities. It also means that the identity is like a "fix" that is desperately needed to maintain an illusion of okay-ness. Indeed, it often takes people several hours to let go of their worker identity after they leave the office. A person may even "need" alcohol or some other drug to step out of the stress of that identity.

Often, in case of workaholics the work itself, or admiration gained by doing all the work, is the drug or "fix." For therapists, the common "identity drug" is the role of being the helper or the knower or the solver. Needless to say, fame, money, or even love from another can be an identity drug. Try to take such an identity away "cold turkey," and the person will fight fiercely to preserve it. He believes he *is* the identity, the role. The trance-like narrowed focus of attention thus causes a loss of the self behind the role, and with that loss, tremendous personal discomfort and/or psychosomatic symptoms.

I worked with a woman who was very attached to her identity as a business woman. Once she became aware of that attachment, she noticed how difficult it was for her to put it down. When she went to the gym for her daily workout, for example, she realized how much she carried her business identity around with her. For some reason, she was very uncomfortable being just one more person working out.

As we worked with the business trance, it became clear that it functioned as an oppositional identity by covering her strong feelings of discomfort with her body. As a child she had suffered a lot of embarrassment, humiliation, and name-calling for her weight problem. She felt that she looked "dumb and stupid" because of her size. She was very bright, however, and found some relief for the dumb-and-stupid identity that infused her body image by getting good grades and being smart. As an adult, the trance identity of dumb and stupid would become active whenever her weight fluctuated, at which point her need to assert her work identity would become very strong.

These different trance identities work in tandem and are so interlocked that they must be processed as a unit. You cannot approach the problem with a goal of, "Let's get rid of the 'dumb-and-stupid' identity."

Self-image identities reflect our core beliefs about our performance and worth as a person: *I am slow; I am inferior; I'm no good; I am an achiever; I'm a loser no matter how hard I try.* These self-image identities are almost always formed early in childhood, primarily as a result of parental influences. Whenever the identity is "negative" or uncomfortable, the child also forms a compensatory *oppositional identity: I'm a fast learner; I am superior to most people; I'm a good girl; I'm easy-going; I'm a winner no matter what.*

As an example, let's say a child is told by his mother: "No, you don't understand." In a state of confusion from the reprimand, the child shifts and narrows his attention, creating an identity called "I-don't-understand." This is followed by the creation of a compensatory identity called "I-*must*-understand." Since both identities exist as a unit, a kind of psychological paralysis takes place in which the "I-don't-understand" identity is held as the generating context or reference point of the "I-*must*-understand" identity. Psychotherapy sessions are filled with the identity binds of people who are driven to succeed in one area or another, yet when they do, they still feel badly. This is because the underlying identity is not recognized or engaged; *both identities must be worked with, simultaneously, as a unit.*

Let's return to our earlier descriptions of trance states in relation to this concept of identities as trances.

First we noted that *trance is characterized by a narrowing, shrinking, or fixating of attention* (Erickson & Rossi, 1976/1980):

> Trance is a condition wherein there is a reduction of the patient's foci of attention to a few inner realities; consciousness has been fixated and focused to a relatively narrow frame of attention rather than being diffused over a broad area. (p. 448)

When we are attached to our identities of role ("I am a mother"), career/job ("I am a dancer"), self-image ("I am a loser"), or oppositional ("I must succeed"), our attention is certainly reduced to those few inner realities that define the identity. We are fixated and focused on a fairly narrow range of experience "rather than being diffused over a broad area."

Furthermore, these identities have boundaries to them—but the *being* does not. This means that in order for you, the being, to take on an identity, you must take on the corresponding boundaries and limitations. Once you fuse with the "boundaried" state and believe that "This is me," you experience all the thoughts, feelings, emotions, and sensations of that limited state/identity. (Without elaborating further, in esoteric literature these boundaried identities are appropriately called "thought-forms.")

The second core characteristic we noted is *the experience of trance as happening to the person*: "Hypnotic response. . .is an expression of behavioral potentials that are experienced as taking place autonomously" (Erickson & Rossi, 1979, p. 4).

Certainly our immersion in our various identities and roles is experienced as on ongoing autonomous process (even archetypal, at times) whereby we feel ourselves as if carried down a stream of expected responses and behaviors. Mothers have one list of expected qualities and duties; stepfathers another. Even the identity of "I am a loser" has quite specific behavioral qualities that appear to the individual to be beyond his or her control.

Finally, we saw *trance as characterized by the spontaneous emergence of various hypnotic phenomena* (Erickson & Rossi, 1976/1980):

> [Trance] is a way of de-automatizing an individual's habitual modes of functioning so that dissociation and many of its attendant classical hypnotic phenomena (e.g., age regression, amnesia, sensory-perceptual distortions, catalepsies, etc.) are frequently manifest in an entirely spontaneous manner. (p. 448)

We have seen (and, for most of us, personally experienced) how trance identities "are frequently manifest in an entirely spontaneous manner."

The one element all the different trance identities have in common is the *you* behind them. There is always a "larger self" behind any kind of creation, be it physical, emotional, psychological, or spiritual. It is very easy to lose track of this awareness when caught up in an identity. If you say, "I have a part inside that wants to win approval, and I also have a part that just wants to be me," you are well describing your oppositional identities. In addition, you are implying the larger self behind the statements with the phrase "I have a part." If you said, "I have a pen," you would never then proceed to identify yourself with the pen. The pen is something *you* have; you are larger than the pen.

The same principle applies with hypnotic identities, except both the *haver* and the *havee* are within you. Typically, we believe that what we are experiencing defines who we are, when in fact we remain senior to and greater than whatever experience we are *having*. Initially, the experience of identity formation is a *creative* process whereby you create the trance and identity you decide will handle the upcoming situation. Again, unfortunately, the identities then *become* an automatic process as they are called upon repeatedly. The task for the therapist is to de-hypnotize the client out of the identity so that the *self* can be experienced as the creative source.

This notion of separation between parts of ourselves is reinforced in the Ericksonian literature, where the unconscious mind is viewed as a separate entity from the conscious mind. In fact, the conscious mind usually receives the bad rap as the part that undermines the healing resources stored in the unconscious mind.

In my view, there really is no such thing as an unconscious mind. There is a *being* who chooses not to remember certain things while choosing to remember others. As mentioned earlier, for me the mind, metaphorically, is like a darkened library. I, the individual who has the mind, walk in with my flashlight and decide where I want to put the light. Where do I want to put my awareness? What do I want to know about?

Grasping this notion of the "you behind the trance" is the corridor to the no-trance state of expanded awareness, where *who you are* remains a fluid and ongoing experience. Entrance to the corridor is gained by becoming familiar with the process of picking up and putting down identities and roles, by beginning to experience a new psychological limberness and flexibility.

Volumes of literature exist in the area of object relations theory concerning the creation of "false selves" that operate autonomously. The "true self," from my point of view, is that which created these false selves.

Treatment of Hypnotic Identities

(1) Ask the client (or proceed alone) to create a three-dimensional picture of the oppositional identities at issue. See them as a hologram, floating in space in full view. Remember that these identities have opposite goals: For example, "I'm stupid" actually has the goal of being stupid; its opposite, "I have to prove that I'm smart," obviously has an opposite goal.

Say the presenting problem is expressed as: "I am so driven to *understand* everything, I drive myself and everybody else crazy. I always feel like I have to know everything, even when it is completely irrelevant." This constitutes an oppositional identity created in compensation for the underlying one of "I don't understand. . .I'm dumb."

Now the person—the being behind the identities—is viewing the two identities. This is usually a person's first experience of separation from or being larger than the problem.

(2) Reminding the client that she is the observer of the two opposing identities, ask her to shift her experience between the two: first becoming one identity—feeling it, being it, as she has done

thousands of times before—and then shift to its opposition—feel it, be it, and then "un-be" it.

(3) Now ask the client to go "inside" and generate a resource for Identity #1 and another resource for Identity #2. Focusing on Identity #1, "I-*must*-understand," the client gets an image of a bird soaring high and free. Next, ask the client to see the bird in a particular part of her body. Perhaps she responds with, "I see the image in my throat."

After letting her quietly experience the integration of the image with her body and Identity #1, ask her to shift her focus to the second identity, "I-don't-understand. . .I'm-dumb," and retrieve a resource the identity could use. After a few moments of inner search, she might respond, "I see a white, fluffy lamb in my stomach." Allow time for a similar integration.

(4) Now ask the client to develop a resource for the identity-free space—the space within her that is not occupied by either identity, a space that feels pure and unlabeled—the observer. This request usually generates images that might be described as spiritual: rainbows, comets, white lights, golden pots, shimmering water, a majestic Himalayan mountain, and so forth. Again, request that the image be placed in any part of the body.

(5) In order to create a sense of overall integration between the two identities, the image resources, and the identity-free space, ask the client to create a resource for the body that allows it to "hold" all this work. The body is the receptacle, the "alchemical pot" in which these different elements merge and transform. Asking the client to create a "holding resource" helps to further ground and integrate the transformations. This begins the process of expanding the context, as discussed in Chapter 6.

(6) Continuing the process of expanding the context is accomplished by asking the client to develop a resource for her social network. She can either imagine a person or persons, or she can use the therapist as a representative. The image comes into her mind—say, it is the trunk of a giant Redwood tree—and she visualizes it within herself and within the therapist or her imagined friends, all simultaneously.

(7) The final step is one of interweaving. Each step represents a strand; at this point all six strands must be woven into a unity. Using hypnotic suggestion, interweave the resources from the two

identities, the identity-free space, the body, and the social network. The important points to remember are:

(a) Make sure that the client is clear about the two identities and has them both floating in space.

(b) Have the client shift into and become each identity, and then shift out the identity several times. This repetitious shifting in and out gives the client the experience of being *more than* the identities.

(c) Make sure the client has retrieved whatever resources are needed for experiencing each identity. Ideally, have the client retrieve a resource from the witness or observer, the body, and the social network while being in the point of view of each.

(d) Interweave each symbolic resource into a unified whole.

(e) After the session is over, give the client a homework assignment to develop an image or symbol of the integrated whole. Most importantly, have the client imagine that the people he or she interacts with also carry a duplicate image or symbol in their bodies.

This approach integrates all aspects of oppositional identities, along with their corresponding contexts and resources. Initially the client is asked to explore identities and resources in a "conscious and unconscious" way. Ultimately, the client comes to understand that he or she has created the identities and the corresponding resources that are then integrated in a no-trance or natural state.

20

The Organizing Principle

THE ORGANIZING PRINCIPLE is a central constellation of *core beliefs*—the hub of our intrapersonal wheel—out of which all life experience radiates. Reinforced countless times as the child grows into the adult, the Organizing Principle functions as a window through which "reality" is viewed, to the exclusion of all other perspectives. Out of our core beliefs come various symptoms. Superimposed over all of them, like a gossamer net, are the Deep Trance Phenomena that hold the Organizing Principle and its symptom structures in place over time.

I have saved this chapter for last because the concept is the subject of another whole book. For now, I will describe the essence of the Organizing Principle only to complete the "puzzle" of symptomatology as it is sustained in a timeless state by Deep Trance Phenomena.

Let me start with an example. Visualize a symptom as a pie of psychodynamic factors. At the center of the pie is a core set of beliefs, the Organizing Principle, that determines the shape, size, color, texture, and outcome of the pie. Say the core belief is, "Life is painful and bitter." Subsets of this core belief would flow into more specific beliefs: "Nothing I do works," "I'll never get ahead," "Bad things just come my way," and so on. Streaming out to form slices of this pie are various symptom structures that manifest this core set of beliefs. And holding it all together are Deep Trance Phenomena—such as age regression, posthypnotic suggestion, pseudo-orientation in time, dissociation, amnesia, etc.—that store the core beliefs in a time-frozen state, keeping them ever-present in the moment, even as time moves forward and years turn into decades.

Our lifestyle is a reflection of our core set of beliefs, our very own Organizing Principle, that is the ultimate coalescence of individual and environment. The Organizing Principle, invisible as it is, nonetheless dominates every aspect of our lives and produces:

(1) *behavioral inevitabilities* comprised of a belief that, for example, "Relationships don't work" and manifested by behavior that ensures negative outcomes;

(2) *emotional inevitabilities* comprised of some belief that "Every time I care for someone I get hurt" and manifested by repeated patterns of feeling abandoned and devastated;

(3) *lifestyle inevitabilities* generated by a belief that, for example, "It's impossible to get ahead" and manifested by job and career failures and a steady income of $5.00 an hour; and

(4) implications of apparent destiny supported by a belief that "I'm not worth anything because I have bad karma" (or because I hated my baby sister when I was a child, or for any reason the person attaches to) and manifested by a consistent and tenacious pattern of self-defeating actions and experiences that spans the individual's lifetime.

As you work with Deep Trance Phenomena in your clients and yourself, you come closer and closer to the underlying Organizing Principle. Often, changing the trances that hold the symptom structures together will have a cybernetic effect, impacting the deeper, more primary Organizing Principle. Such work must proceed slowly and cautiously. In yogic literature, continual references are made to "untying the knot of the heart." In our contemporary terms this is synonymous with the process of identifying the individual's Organizing Principle and then slowly changing it. As you begin to untie the knots (the beliefs)—and the symptoms and trances that keep them ever-present—you are, in essence, untying a portion of the person's world view—one's very reference point to physical life.

To successfully untie the "knot of the heart"—the Organizing Principle—frees the person from living in ever-changing trance states and points the way toward a quantum leap in personal evolution. To experience this leap requires a kind of psycho-emotional death in which the old foundation is completely removed. In other words, the "I" that believes that "Life is painful and bitter" dies or dissolves and a new "I," free of symptoms and limiting trance states, is formed. The person begins to allow an ever expanding awareness that includes in its embrace the jewels of human life: new experiences of compassion, love, and oneness.

Epilogue

Foundations of Quantum Psychology

As we bring *Trances People Live* to a close, three concluding issues remain important. First, how do Deep Trance Phenomena relate to Quantum Physics in general and to Quantum Psychology in particular? Second, if hypnotic phenomena are self-created, what are the implications for the specialty of hypnosis and the entire field of psychotherapy? Third, using *Trances People Live* as a gradient step, what is the future of psychology in relation to the new knowledge available to us from Quantum Physics? What techniques and approaches must be developed to facilitate a corresponding paradigmatic shift in psychotherapy, its theory and practice?

Let us begin with the first point. Few therapists would deny that using similar techniques in working with different clients does not yield similar results. In modern psychotherapy, what is emphasized is the application of a particular technique to a particular psychodynamic problem. This emphasis ignores the individual, the being, the you behind the symptom. Quantum Physics has filled this gap by demonstrating the influential and deterministic role of the observer behind and beyond the experiment. Applying this insight to psychotherapy would mean that therapists turn their focus away from resolving the problem and onto the person (observer) who is creating the reality defined as a problem.

If problems are intrapersonal and self-generated, where does this leave hypnosis and psychotherapy? Although all problems are ultimately intrapersonal (self-to-self), they occur in an interpersonal context. This contextual relationship places hypnosis and psychotherapy at the doorway of a new model. The old model tends to objectify the client, excluding him or her as the observer or knower or being that generates the current reality. Our next leap is to "know the knower" or explore the being, the individual, who is the creative life force behind each of our perceptual frameworks— frameworks that create our subjective experiences and limit our "beinghood" to much less then its full potential. Moving through this doorway and allowing the "being behind the problem" to be explored is, I hope, the new direction of psychology.

The birth of psychotherapy by Sigmund Freud at the turn of the century had its scientific basis in Newtonian Physics, which contended that the world was mechanistic in nature and could be objectively measured. Only with Albert Einstein's discovery of relativity theory—that measurement was dependent upon the relative speed and position of what was being measured—did the paradigm begin to shift. It is important to note that although Einstein was a major contributor to the development of Quantum Mechanics, he himself found it difficult to accept the results of his own research. In the now famous Copenhagen debates between Einstein and Neils Bohr, Einstein argued against the major principles of Quantum Physics.

Trances People Live: Healing Approaches In Quantum Psychology is a gradient bridging the psychological implications of Newtonian Physics with the psychological implications of the new Quantum Physics. Since we are pointing the way from self-created trance states to Quantum Psychology, I will briefly outline the four major tenets of Quantum Psychology, based directly on principles from the field of Quantum Physics (Herbert, 1985):

(1) The observer influences his observed reality.
Werner Heisenberg

Reality is created by observation. There is no reality in absence of observation.

Copenhagen Interpretation (Part II)

(2) Everything interpenetrates everything else. Reality is an undivided wholeness.

David Bohm

(3) Everything is made of emptiness; form is condensed emptiness.

Albert Einstein

(4) There are no local causes. Reality itself is non-local.

John Stewart Bell

For now, we stand on the beginning foundation of understanding the first principle in relation to the Deep Trance Phenomena that serve as our observer-created medium. In my forthcoming book, *Quantum Consciousness: The Discovery and Birth of Quantum Psychology: The Physics of Consciousness*, I will explore all of these principles in terms of their psychological implications and applications as we begin to make the shift from Newtonian Psychology to Quantum Psychology.

Appendix I

Stripping Gears: Deconstructing Phobic Responses

*E*RICKSON has described several ingenious methods of treating phobias that involve the principles of utilization, reframing, reinterpretation, and progressive diminution (Erickson & Rossi, 1979; Rossi & Ryan, 1985; Rossi, Ryan & Sharp, 1983). Reading case reports of his work with phobic patients is always inspiring, thanks to Erickson's utterly creative and original solutions.

Integrating elements of Erickson's treatment of phobias with my own concepts of Deep Trance Phenomena, I developed a technique, which I named "stripping gears," that has been quite successful.

Step 1: Allow the Deep Trance Phenomena to reach fruition. As in our previous Deep Trance work, ask the client to visualize her phobic response at its peak (in an airplane, elevator, tall building, or wherever). Note any minimal body cues of muscle tightness and shallow breathing.

Step 2: Interrupt the self-to-self trance by adding an interpersonal context. Ask the client to breathe and look at you while she consciously continues to tighten her muscles in the process of re-creating her fear.

Step 3: "Strip the gears" by adding a positive resource. At the peak or apex of the fear response ask the client, "What was your favorite kind of play when you were a child?" At first the client feels a sense of disruption and confusion as the conscious mind begins to remember the pleasurable activity, while the unconscious mind is still holding on to the old emotional response. Suddenly, body tightness is reassociated with a pleasant memory. There is a mental clash, a sense of "non-compute," as the phobic pattern is thrown off its usual course. This is equivalent to "stripping gears" in a car: the car (the phobic response) is headed forward at full throttle, 60 mph, when it is suddenly thrown into reverse. As a result, the transmission (the patterned response) falls out!

Step 4: Interweave the phobic response with positive resources. Using metaphors, analogies, and sensory imagery, the therapist takes the newly dislodged and splintered phobic response and weaves it into the fabric of the client's inner, experiential resources. This ensures a thorough integration of the new learning, leaving "no lose threads." Following is a sample of this interweaving process:

A woman I was working with complained of an airplane phobia. I asked her to duplicate her phobia as she breathed and looked at me, and at the peak of her phobic feelings, I asked her: "What was your favorite thing to do as a child?" She responded, "Playing with the leaves." I continued:

"There are leaves of the trees, and a little girl, and how nice it is to play in the leaves, a girl playing in the leaves of the trees. And that terrible airplane, how awful it is. I don't want to get on leaves of a tree. And an airplane can look like a leaf or a leave, and it's nice to know you can. . .leave the leaves and the airplane, you leave for work in the morning, and I don't have to tell you that an airplane leaves to go to faraway places, races, traces of smoke from an airplane. . .can. . .leave a little girl or even a self feeling really comfortable."

In this way new associations within the context of the phobia are being created. In addition the pleasant sensations of the little girl with her leaves are blended with the tightening of muscles in the airplane.

Appendix II

Utilizing Archetypes

WHEN A CLIENT'S material is reframed in an archetypal context, it is possible to move from the personal, content-oriented level to a transpersonal, process-oriented level. Often, severe abuse experienced in childhood will block the therapeutic process and the client remains unable to resolve his current problems and symptoms. When the client does not appear to possess the ego strength to confront the material as it is manifested in symptomatic trance phenomena, the therapist can make a clinical judgment to make use of archetypes (Jung, 1959) as a means of helping the client to create a new relationship.

The Mother Archetype

I worked with one woman whose mother, a moody alcoholic, had just died. Consequently, the past relationship and current grief presented much unfinished business for the client, now 38.

Using her natural state of trance, I began to differentiate between her birth mother and the archetypal mother. Actually, first I got an image of the moon, which I followed. I talked in trance about the different phases of the moon—the new moon, the half moon, the sliver moon—and how each phase has its own emotional impact. The moon mother and the birth mother share some of these changing characteristics, but the moon mother is omnipresent (because she is within, in a self-to-self relationship).

I continued to develop and deepen the therapeutic qualities of the moon mother as contrasted with the qualities of the birth mother, who is really the vehicle of the larger archetypal experience. This differentiation created clear and distinct boundaries for the client. It helped her view her birth mother in a different perspective, as she drew on the compassion and unconditional acceptance of the moon mother.

Five points need to be discussed here. First, this woman was an astrologer, so using the moon was a way of differentiating metaphorically different aspects of her mother's personality. Second, in India the moon is regarded as an aspect of the archetypal mother; this particular client had studied meditation and was interested in these abstractions. Third, because of the mother's alcoholism, my client had fused her mother with the archetype of the universal mother; this, too, needed to be differentiated.

Finally, since she was an adult-child of an alcoholic, I planned to suggest she attend a 12-step program. These programs make use of a "higher power." Often, however, adult-children of alcoholics or incest survivors fuse their parents with God or the higher power. This "transpersonal transference" had to be shifted in order for her to continue her recovery.

I cannot overemphasize the importance of using archetypes and metaphors that reflect the client's frame of reference; otherwise, at some level the client will not accept the reframe that is being offered.

The Snake Archetype

In another more severe case, my client was hallucinating snakes coming out of her mouth, ears, and nose. I knew that she had experienced incidents of sexual molestation as a child, including multiple experiences of forced oral sex with her stepfather. I proceeded with great caution.

In trance, I asked her if she could push the snakes out of her mouth. She showed signs of age regression and answered slowly that if she did push the snakes out, she would die. I realized that the intensity of her traumas exceeded her capacity to enter the space represented by the snakes, so I hypnotically projected her into the future (using pseudo-orientation in time) to a time when this experience was resolved. She spontaneously visualized the archetypal image of the snake moving up her spine, which I reinforced by talking about the Kundalini shakti from the base of the spine through the crown of the head and how it was considered a pathway to enlightenment. I then spent an hour and a half going through each movement of the snake up her spine and integrating this "future" experience into the present moment. Conceptually, I reframed the frightening image of the writhing snakes into a positive one in which they were merely seeking their way home (their pathway up the spine).

Utilizing the Deep Trance Phenomenon of pseudo-orientation in time had created a context for the emergence of a healing archetypal image—which, as the therapist, I could have in no way planned or strategically plotted. It was an unexpected confluence of dynamics that I find comes naturally when the process stays focused in the present moment. This means that interaction between client and therapist remains flowing and alive rather than rigidified in preplanned interventions or codified in preordained values about the "right way" to do therapy.

I do not wish to imply that I ignored or discounted her sexual abuse. Quite to the contrary, these types of experiences must be explored and experienced in various ways. The purpose of this particular session was to alleviate the snake hallucinations first before exploring her symptomatic Deep Trance Phenomena.

The Archetype of the "Seeker"

In working with an alcoholic, I reframed the client's experience from that of being a fighter, fending off the impulses of alcoholism, to that of being a seeker in search of a spiritual connection that was free of pain. He had used alcohol to seek an experience of life that he felt was unattainable—one that was painless. He was seeking a transcendental experience of "no pain." Instead of looking inward for his spiritual roots, he was looking outward to the alcohol to give him the solace.

My task was to work hypnotically to assist him in creating the inner reality of "seeker"—to tap into his inner essence of striving for connection to a higher power. In trance I talked about the archetypal seeker as one whose character is strongly motivated toward finding "his inner power"—yet the seeker typically begins his journey in a flawed state. The powerful phrase, "the dark night of the soul," refers to a seeker about to turn toward a pathway of light. Now, instead of fighting alcohol, he could begin to seek within himself.

Obviously, supplying one archetypal image does not undo decades of alcoholic behavior, but this image was a powerful one for the client, and it worked on him over a period of several months. He gradually understood the profound difference between focusing his energy on battling alcoholism, versus focusing his energy on seeking his own spirituality. He did not stop drinking "cold turkey," but steadily tapered off as other, more healthful desires began to surface. Furthermore, this process facilitated and reinforced his work in Alcoholics Anonymous by helping to increase his interest in seeking the "higher power" as well as developing the inner seeker within himself.

It is important to stress that the therapist cannot really "plan" to use archetypal imagery. The direction toward this level of working comes from the client's cues that personal resources are scarce and ego strength is limited. The Deep Trance Phenomena that are holding the symptom in place can be directly addressed as one develops an archetypal reframe.

In conclusion, symptoms and problems can be approached through various levels of abstraction, when needed. If change cannot be effected through the conscious mind, then the therapist turns to the unconscious for resources; if none are forthcoming, the therapist can move still further into the collective unconscious in search of resources that will shift the client's subjective experience of the problem state.

Appendix III

"Zigzagging": Integrating Traumatic Experience

AS MENTIONED in Appendix II, there are times when an individual's attachment to past trauma is so strong that the content must be addressed in some way. Therefore, before beginning work on the Deep Trance Phenomena that are holding the current symptom in place (as well as the original trauma), I might use the "jigsaw" technique developed by Erickson (which I call "zigzagging") whereby the affective and cognitive elements of an early trauma are experienced separately.

Erickson described his ingenious method of helping a medical student retrieve a trauma blanketed by amnesia in a 1955 article entitled, "Self-Exploration in the Hypnotic State" (Erickson, 1955/1980). The student first began reliving affective elements of the trauma on an unconscious level, stating in trance, "It's too big, I can't do it. Tell me how." Erickson's response was: "I can't tell you how, but I can offer a suggestion. You say it's too big. Why not do it a part here, a part there, instead of the whole thing at once, and then puts the parts together into the whole big thing?" (p. 431).

The student continued to relive intense emotional aspects of the trauma on an unconscious level. Coming out of trance, the student asked to recall the trauma consciously. Since this hypnotic work was being done in a teaching setting with other medical students, Erickson explored a variety of concerns with his audience:

> As for the method of achieving a conscious understanding, there were certain considerations he [the subject] should have in mind. Would he want the whole thing to irrupt into his conscious mind all at once? Or would he prefer to have it come piecemeal, one part at a time, with the possibility of halting the process and mustering his strength so that he could more easily endure the next development. *Would he want to separate the affective from the cognitive elements and experience the one or the other first?* (p. 433)

Here Erickson is careful to give ask the subject how *he* wants to recover his trauma. Erickson does not make any assumptions about how to proceed. The subject opts for the piecemeal approach, and Erickson obliges by helping him zigzag back and forth between emotion and content. By the end of the session all the "pieces" of the traumatic puzzle had been assembled, but at a pace that was digestible for the subject.

In summarizing his jigsaw approach, Erickson explains (Erickson & Rossi, 1981):

> Hypnosis can also allow you to divide up your patient's problems. For example, a patient comes to you with some traumatic experience in the past which has resulted in a phobic reaction or an anxiety state. One can put him in a deep trance and suggest that he recover only the emotional aspects of that experience. . . .In other words, one can split off the intellectual aspects of a problem for a patient and leave only the emotional aspects to be dealt with. One can have a patient cry out very thoroughly over the emotional aspects of a traumatic experience and then later let him recover it in a jigsaw fashion—that is, let him recover a little bit of the intellectual content of the traumatic experience of the past, then a little bit of the emotional content—and these different aspects need not necessarily be connected. Thus, you let the young medical student see the pitchfork, then you let him feel the pain he experiences in the gluteal

region, then you let him see the color green, then you let him feel himself stiff and rigid, and then you let him feel the full horror of his stiffness and rigidity. *Various bits of the incident recovered in this jigsaw fashion allow you to eventually recover an entire, forgotten traumatic experience of childhood that had been governing this person's behavior in medical school and handicapping his life very seriously.* (pp. 6-7) [Italics added]

Any therapist making use of Erickson's therapeutic creations must integrate them with his or her own style or context. In this case, I have added two elements that represent basic principles of my work.

Step 1: Help the client develop a state of objective witnessing. Before returning to the trauma via age-regression, the therapist helps the client experience a new way of observing. Rather than withdrawing through dissociation (which is a defense mechanism), the client learns to observe in a detached but *present* manner. In Buddhist writings, this is called "mindfulness." Dissociation happens automatically; witnessing happens only through the conscious choice of the client.

In teaching the client how to witness, I usually suggest that he begin to visualize the trauma as though it were floating in a very distant bubble or cloud. Then, as feelings or thoughts begin to surface, they are injected into the distant bubble. The client "practices" this procedure until he becomes accustomed to the sensation or experience of detaching from an emerging emotion and observing it "out there."

Step 2: The therapist becomes the "marker" of present time. To add a constant point of stability and present focus, the therapist asks the client to select some physical characteristic about the therapist that will differentiate him from the past trauma being relived. This differentiation accomplishes two important therapeutic goals: (1) the therapist can represent the client's present, with all its lifetime of resources, which far exceed what was available during the actual trauma; and (2) the illusion of being accompanied and supported is created—as Erickson did so masterfully when he acted as the

"February Man" (Erickson & Rossi, 1989). The therapist both marks and anchors the present and simultaneously accompanies the client back in time.

This step is particularly useful when working with incest survivors of the opposite sex. When working with female clients with past sexual traumas, I have found it is important to differentiate myself from the field of men so that I am not converted into the perpetrator during deep trance work. I might ask a client, "As you look at me now, what about me—my beard, my glasses, the rings on my fingers—can remind you that I am Stephen and it is 1987?" Throughout the age-regressed trance work, I then remind the client, "As you look at my glasses (or whatever item she picked), you know that I am Stephen, and that it is 1987." This helps to curtail the projection and transference so easily activated in this kind of work.

Step 3: Zigzag the content and the emotional component back and forth. This is Erickson at his best: separating thinking from feeling, separating an experience from one's reaction to the experience. You begin by suggesting that the client re-experience a small portion of the event without feeling any emotional response to it. Once this portion of the content has been expressed and an amnesia induced, you suggest that she now experience the emotion of that portion, without remembering the content. By zigzagging back and forth between digestible pieces of the experience, each time pushing back the boundary of the repressed trauma, the entire event can be integrated without disrupting the equilibrium or integrity of the client.

References

Aitken, R. (1978). *A Zen Wave*. Tokyo: Weatherhill.

Erickson, M. (1952/1980). Deep hypnosis and its induction. In E. Rossi (Ed.), *The Collected Papers of Milton H. Erickson on Hypnosis. I. The Nature of Hypnosis and Suggestion* (pp. 139-167. New York: Irvington.

Erickson, M. (1955/1980). Self-exploration in the hypnotic state. In E. Rossi (Ed.), *The Collected Papers of Milton H. Erickson on Hypnosis. Vol IV. Innovative Hypnotherapy* (pp. 427-436). New York: Irvington.

Erickson, M. (1967/1980). Further experimental investigation of hypnosis: Hypnotic and nonhypnotic realities. In E. Rossi (Ed.), *The Collected Papers of Milton H. Erickson on Hypnosis. I. The Nature of Hypnosis and Suggestion* (pp. 18-82). New York: Irvington.

Erickson, M. (1980). Age regression: Two unpublished fragments of a student's study. In E. Rossi (Ed.), *The Collected Papers of Milton H. Erickson on Hypnosis. Vol. III. Hypnotic Investigation of Psychodynamic Processes* (pp.104-111). New York: Irvington.

Erickson, M., & Rossi, E. (1976/1980). Two-level communication and the microdynamics of trance. In E. Rossi (Ed.), *The Collected Papers of Milton H. Erickson on Hypnosis I. The Nature of Hypnosis and Suggestion* (pp. 430-451). New York: Irvington.

Erickson, M., & Rossi, E. (1977/1980). Autohypnotic experiences of Milton H. Erickson. In E. Rossi (Ed.), *The Collected Papers of Milton H. Erickson on Hypnosis. I. The Nature of Hypnosis and Suggestion* (pp. 108-132). New York:

Erickson, M., & Rossi, E. (1979). *Hypnotherapy: An Exploratory Casebook.* New York: Irvington.

Erickson, M., & Rossi, E. (1981). *Experiencing Hypnosis: Therapeutic Approaches to Altered States.* New York: Irvington.

Erickson, M., & Rossi, E. (1989). *The February Man: Evolving Consciousness and Identity in Hypnotherapy.* New York: Brunner/Mazel.

Erickson, M., Rossi, E., & Rossi, S. (1976). *Hypnotic Realities.* New York: Irvington.

Gilligan, S. (1987). *Therapeutic Trances: The Cooperation Principle in Ericksonian Hypnotherapy.* New York: Brunner/Mazel.

Herbert, N. (1985). *Quantum Reality: Beyond the New Physics.* New York: Anchor Press, Doubleday.

Horner, J. (1988). Private conversation.

Jnaneshvari: A Song Sermon of the Bhagavad Gita, Vol II. (1962). Translated by V. G. Pradhan. Bombay, India: Blackie & Son Publishers. (Orginally published in England in 1948.)

Jung, C. (1959). *Archetypes of the Collective Unconscious. Vol. 9(1). The Collected Works of C. G. Jung.* Translated by R.F.C. Hull. Bollingen Series XX. Princeton, New Jersey: Princeton University Press.

Lao Tzu. (1958). Quoted in Fung Yu-Lan, *A Short History of Chinese Philosophy.* New York: Macmillan.

Rossi, E. (1986). *The Psychobiology of Mind-Body Healing: New Concepts of Therapeutic Hypnosis.* New York: W. W. Norton.

Rossi, E., & Ryan, M. (Eds.) (1986). *Mind-Body Communication in Hypnosis. Vol. 3. The Seminars, Workshops, and Lectures of Milton H. Erickson.* New York: Irvington.

Rossi, E., Ryan, M., & Sharp, F. (Eds.) (1984). *Healing in Hypnosis. Vol. 1. The Seminars, Workshops, and Lectures of Milton H. Erickson.* New York: Irvington.

Rossi, E., & Ryan, M. (Eds.) (1991). *Creative Choice in Hypnosis. Vol. IV. The Seminars, Workshops and Lectures of Milton H. Erickson.* New York: Irvington.

Fagan, J., & Shepherd, I. (Eds.). (1970). *Gestalt Therapy Now*. New York: Harper & Row.

Singh, J. (1979), *Vijnanabhairava or Divine Consciousness*. Delhi, India: Motilal Bangrsidas.

Tart, C. (1987). Aikido and the concept of ki. *Psychological Perspectives, 18*(2), 332-348.

Whitaker, C. (1989). *Midnight Musings of a Family Therapist*. New York: W. W. Norton.

Whitaker, C., & Malone, T. (1987). *The Roots of Psychotherapy*. New York: Brunner/Mazel.

Wolinsky, S. (1992). *Quantum Consciousness: The Discovery and Birth of Quantum Psychology: The Physics of Consciousness*.

Wolf, F. (1981). *Taking the Quantum Leap*. New York: Harper & Row.

Wu Wei. (1967). *The I Ching or Book of Changes*. Translated by R. Wilhelm. Princeton: Princeton University Press.

Yampolski, P. (Trans.) (1971). *The Zen Master Hakuin: Selected Writings*. New York: Columbia University Press.

Index*

---

*Major headings for each Deep Trance Phenomenon are in bold-face type.

Anesthesia
  "beach trance" and 12, 14
  Ericksonian approaches to 203-
    204
  pain and 203, 205
Anorexia-bulimia 36-37, 55
Anxiety
  Deep Trance Phenomena and 6-
    7, 32, 99, 100-102
Archetypes 239-242
  mother 239-240
  seeker 241-242
  snake 240-241
Arjuna 61
Attention, narrowing of
  anxiety and 32
  confusion and 166
  differentiation and (*see also*
    separate listing) 149
  feelings and 41
  fusion and 49, 218
  hypnotic identities and 218
  identification and 49
  misidentification and 58, 59
  meditation and 40, 42, 44, 46
  mundane examples of 46-47
  "no-trance" and 46, 48
  pain 203, 207
  paradox and 43-49
  reactions as 15-16, 81-82
  symptomatic trance as 31-32, 56
  time distortion and 179
  trance as 9-10, 221
  trigger mechanism and 214, 216
  voluntary vs. involuntary 47, 49
Behavioral inevitabilities
  Organizing Principle and 228
  posthypnotic suggestion and
    118, 182, 216
Beliefs, core 227-229
Bell, John Stewart 233
Bioenergetics 177
Body
  amnesia and 134
  confusion and 174
  context and 62-63, 108-109
  dissociation from 107-109, 200-
    201
  as field 62, 63
  hypnotic dreaming and 193, 194
  hypnotic identities and 224-225
  obesity and 201
  self and 63-66
  time and 175-177, 182, 183
  trance and 176, 193
Bohm, David 233

Bohr, Neils 232
Braid, James 131, 135
Breath (breathing)
  "breathe and look at me" 33-37,
    64-66, 87, 88, 89, 99, 100,
    113, 134, 190, 191, 194,
    200, 206, 236
  confusion and 173
  dissociation and 64
  expanded awareness and 64
  interrupting trance states 33-37,
    64
  selfhood and 64
  symptoms and 34
Checkerboard Technique 151
Cheek, David 135
"Child within" 185-187, 192-193, 195
Choice 7, 60-61, 62, 115, 123-126,
    137, 175, 176, 187, 189,
    192-193, 216
Co-dependency 96, 156, 177-178
Complexes 132
Confusion 165-174
  abuse and 172
  allowing 171, 172-173
  attention in 166
  body, grounding in 174
  breath and 173
  contexts of 168-171, 173
  differentiation of 173
  fusion and 172
  hypnotic and oppositional
    identities and 165-168, 171,
    172
  interpersonal 169-170
  origins of 166
  posthypnotic suggestion and
    129-130
  projection and 167, 168, 172
  resistance to 165, 166
  self-generated 170-171
  symbols of 173-174
  task and object-oriented 169
  therapists and 171
  treatment of 172-174
  witnessing 173
Content vs. process 21-28, 243-246
  agoraphobia and 23
  archetypes and 239
  Erickson and 24-28
  "jigsaw" method and 26-28
  molestation and 22
  posthypnotic suggestion and 128
  relationship problems and 23
  time distortion and 179
  unconscious and 25-28